CURE THAT COLD!

FIGHT THAT FLU!

A Do-It-Yourself Guide
To
Homeopathic Treatment

By

Doris Elaine Sauter, M. Div.

Other Books By
Doris Elaine Sauter

Non-Fiction, edited with Gwen Lee

What If Our World Is Their Heaven?
The Final Conversations of Philip K. Dick

Poetry

Prayers From the Other Woman

CURE THAT COLD!

FIGHT THAT FLU!

A Do-It-Yourself Guide
To
Homeopathic Treatment

By

Doris Elaine Sauter, M. Div.

© 2004 Doris Elaine Sauter
An Earlier, Limited Edition Of This Book Was Published As
Cure, Cold! Fly, Flu! © 1998
First Printing September 2004

✝ Divine Mercy Press ✝
1973 Apple Street, #35, Oceanside, California 92054
5319 Willis Avenue, Dallas, Texas 75206

ISBN 0-9755471-4-3

For my sister, Dee Schore

❖ ❖ ❖

"A sister is a gift to the heart, a friend to the spirit, a golden thread to the meaning of life."
—Isadora James

"How do people make it through life without a sister?"
—Sara Corpening

First, Grateful Thanks

Thank you to all my clients in California and Texas, who gave me the experience to write this book. My prayers are for your continued health.

Grateful appreciation to Sara Purcell Perine, Alissa Gould, and Boiron Homeopathic Pharmacy for their research material on Oscillococcinum and homeopathy research in general. Also, the same goes to Matrixx Initiatives, Inc. for the studies concerning Zicam, and to the helpful folks at Kent Homeopathic Associates for their information about computer homeopathy.

Thanks need to go to Dr. Nina Cahan, MD, whose unselfish gift of her time gave me valuable advice on when to see a doctor for colds and flu.

Thanks also go to Lené Oliver and Sean Allen, who gave me much-needed computer advice when the Mac had a tantrum during the final preparation of this book. Gratitude also to Paula Johnston, who at the eleventh hour helped with putting *Cure That Cold!* in its final format. And thanks also need to go to Gene Baird, who rescued me from Computer Hell many times, and who met my interruptions with good humor in spite of his demanding job.

Many thanks to Cathy Arthur, a great editor and an even better friend, who edited the first version of this book, as well as to the eagle-eyed Erika Hall, for her careful proofreading of this current edition. Their suggestions for this book were not always followed but were always greatly appreciated. Even more precious to me is their friendship and patience with me.

And, last but not least, to Bekkah Arthur and Muriel Cerf, who graciously let me into their homes (and their bedrooms) to take photos for a possible cover for this book, to the "unknown editor" who wished to remain nameless, to Pat Hildebrand, to lent me a second pair of eyes in the eleventh hour, and to Will Clarke, for his unflagging support and his creation of the final cover for this book.

D. E. S.

Table Of Contents

Preface

Almost everyone—even the healthiest among us—has a cold or flu horror story. A Christmas party missed; a child's wedding suffered through instead of enjoyed; SAT tests performed with mediocre results; the big date that falls flat because of a red nose or sneezing fits. No matter how stoic we try to be, there's no hiding the misery of a cold.

It would be bad enough if our time and energy were the only things robbed from us by a cold or flu; our money is lost as well. Americans spend millions of dollars a year on cold and flu medicines, many of which don't work or, at best, only cover up the symptoms and prolong the illness.

Even if you do bite the bullet and go to a medical doctor, often all he can do is tell you colds aren't fatal and give you a prescription for antibiotics "so that it won't turn into strap throat." An honest doctor will tell you that he has nothing in his arsenal that will cure a cold. Colds are caused by a virus. With time your own immune system will fight it off.

❖ ❖ ❖ ❖ ❖

In my fourteen years practicing and teaching homeopathy, I was never able to find homeopathic texts dedicated to the treatment of colds and flu. Many books will list colds or flu as a subsection, but an in-depth treatment of colds and flu is hard to find. Hence, this book.

Here's what I hope *Cure Colds, Fly Flu!* will do for you:

1. Explain homeopathy in clear terms that you will understand.

2. Provide guidelines for practicing homeopathy safely and effectively in your own home.

3. Give you a working knowledge of over twenty of the most common homeopathic cold and flu remedies.

Are there other remedies for colds and flu that are not included in this book? Most definitely, yes. Under the symptom nasal coryza (which is the homeopathic term for a stuffy nose) there are almost two hundred remedies, any of which might cure your cold immediately. However, although there are two hundred remedies that *might* cure, many of these other remedies are rarely used. I have narrowed down the scope of this book to cover the remedies that, statistically, are the more commonly used cold and flu remedies because they have a higher probability of helping you.

In writing this book I have followed certain homeopathic traditions that require mention. First of all, to preserve the language found in most homeopathic repertories and *Materia Medicas*, I have omitted the prepositions listed under remedy symptoms. For example, a "desire *for* spicy foods" I have shortened to "desires spicy foods." Also, in keeping with Homeopathic history, and colloquial use among homeopaths, I have sometimes treated the remedy as an entity itself. It is common among homeopaths not to say, "The person needing Belladonna is not thirsty," but simply to say, "Belladonna is not thirsty." I hope these conventions will not confuse you. And, in keeping with correct English usage, I have avoided the ubiquitous "they" and used "he" or "she" in referring to a singular person, assuming that you will know that those terms refer to both male and female subjects.

If you do your best to read and understand this book, it is my hope that you will be able to decrease the number of colds and flu you have and shorten the duration of your illness.

Welcome to homeopathy! I hope it is as interesting and exciting to you as it was for me!

Doris Elaine Sauter, M. Div.

Part One:

INTRODUCTION TO

HOMEOPATHY

What Is Homeopathy, Anyway?

The next several chapters are about the history of homeopathy. These chapters will be useful to you if you have friends or family members who are apt to ask questions about homeopathy. What they will provide is a context so that you will be better able to understand the principles and theory of homeopathy and answer their questions about this new method of treatment for your family.

However, if you are afflicted with a cold or flu at this moment and are searching these pages to find help for yourself *now*, please feel free to skip these chapters and go straight to the next section, *Taking Care of Business*. You can always catch up later when you are not sneezing and coughing.

◈　◈　◈　◈　◈

Legend has it that Samuel Hahnemann had a stern father who felt that higher education was a luxury not necessary during hard times. He tried to curtail his son's schooling; Samuel made a candlestick out of clay so he could study at night without his father seeing a metal candlestick missing. Apocryphal or not, this story conveys a truth: Samuel Hahnemann was a born scholar who couldn't live without his studies. Add to this that his father taught him "Never learn or listen passively" and you have the makings of a passionate innovator.

Hahnemann was born in Meissen, Germany, in 1755. Meissen, once renowned for its porcelain, had been devastated by war and the porcelain business fell on hard times. Hahnemann's father had apprenticed him to a shopkeeper in a nearby town, but he ran away, unable to trade scholarship for the life of a merchant. His mother had to hide the boy for a few days while she softened his father to the idea of his coming home.

Hahnemann's father was still adamant about not paying for the boy's education, but Hahnemann's teacher, Professor Muller, seeing promise, paid his tuition for him. He also brought Hahnemann with him when he transferred to a more advanced school. Muller was so impressed with Hahnemann that he put him in charge of other students in the Greek class. He was also accorded special privileges, such as not attending classes in which he already had proficiency.

By the time Hahnemann was ready to pursue college, he had decided to go to medical school. With his excellent grades he could have chosen to go to any medical school he wished. Although was raised a Lutheran, Hahnemann went to a small Catholic hospital to learn under his mentor, Dr. Quarin.

Baron Samuel Von Bruckenthal, the Governor of Transylvania, was impressed with Hahnemann after he entered medical school, and made him librarian of his personal library. This post enabled him to deepen his language proficiency. Sources vary, but they say that Hahnemann was knowledgeable in German, Latin, Greek, English, French, Spanish, Italian, Hebrew, and Arabic by the time he left his post.

Hahnemann received his medical degree in 1779, but by 1789 he had become disenchanted with the field and earned his living doing medical translation and chemistry rather than practicing medicine. Hahnemann was disappointed in current practices, which were more often harmful than helpful.

We tend to think that medicine has always been practiced the way we practice today. But the historical reality is that various schools of medicine prior to the present day were practiced concurrently during Hahnemann's era. There were several popular schools of medicine in Hahnemann's day, all of which employed useless if not destructive means to heal illness. Whatever particular school of medicine a person's physician ascribed to determined what type of care he or she would receive.

The oldest medical system still in use in the late 1700's was that of Asclepiades, a second-century Greek who taught that good health was the balance between tension and relaxation. This school was called Methodism.

Another popular school of medicine was headed by John Brown. Brown was an aspiring professor and theologian who failed at both careers before turning to medicine. He clamed that all diseases were caused by an excess or deficit of nature's stimulation. People who lacked stimulation were called "asthenics" and given stimulants. People who had too much stimulation he called "sthenics" and gave them opium to tone them down. It was said that "Brownism killed more people than the French Revolution and the Napoleonic Wars put together." However, the school was so popular it was not abandoned until late in the nineteenth century.

The Humoral Theory dated from the Middle Ages. It was believed that the cause of all illness was the excess of one of four bodily fluids: blood, black bile, yellow bile, or phlegm. Health was achieved by creating an outlet for the excess humor. Patients were burned, cut, branded, and lanced in order for the fluid to drain out.

Another popular system of medicine was created by Broussais, a surgeon in Napoleon's army who wanted to apply military tactics to the treatment of disease. Some of his ideas were: there is no disease, only symptoms; almost all of mankind's illness stems from inflammation of the digestive tract; the healing power of nature does not exist; and that almost any disease can be cured by starvation and leeches. Nourishment was withheld and leeches were applied to the bodies of the ill to suck out the "diseased blood."

The Humoral Theory and Broussais's theory of the treatment of disease formed the rationale for the most popular treatment of disease in Hahnemann's day. This was bloodletting, and to the physicians it made logical sense. If disease is really caused by an excess of one bodily fluid or another, then ridding the patient of that fluid might cure them. The theory was that bloodletting would only let the bad blood out; good blood would remain, and the patient would thus be cured.

The second most common treatment of illness was polypharmacy, meaning "to use more than one drug at a time." In Hahnemann's day, it was not at all unusual for a patient to be given between sixty-five and four hundred different kinds of medicine in an effort to cure him. These doses were given over a short span of time, the reasoning being that *one* of many must certainly cure.

Hahnemann criticized these standard medical practices. He disagreed that bloodletting only let out the bad blood and not the good. He thought that polypharmacy was a terrible treatment on two counts: first, because it was bad for the patient and, secondly, it made it impossible for the physician to recognize the actions of individual medicines. He also thought the accepted treatment for epidemics such as smallpox and scarlet fever were useless and even harmful.

After Hahnemann's daughter became ill, suffering terribly during standard treatment, his dissatisfaction with medical practice grew; he longed to find an alternative.

Hahnemann was working as a medical translator on Cullen's treatise on fever when he read a passage stating that cinchona bark cured fever because of its bitter and astringent qualities. Hahnemann wondered at this—remember, he never "learned or listened passively"—because there were other bitter and astringent substances that did not cure fever as well as cinchona. Hahnemann took cinchona bark himself and developed a fever with the same qualities of fevers that cinchona bark was famous for curing. Shortly after that, he took a dose of mercury, and developed the same symptoms that a dose of mercury cured. He began to wonder if substances that *caused* certain symptoms could *cure* an illness with those same symptoms as well.

Still not believing, it was the third incident that convinced Hahnemann he was dealing with a scientific truth and not coincidence. He had a friend, a painter, who was fatigued and had become indifferent to his work and to everyone around him. Hahnemann noticed that he had developed the habit of sucking on his brush when he was using sepia-colored ink. He made a remedy from the sepia ink, gave it to the painter, and the painter was cured.

It was then that Hahnemann began to formulate the first law of homeopathy: a substance that can give someone symptoms in a crude or strong dose will cure those symptoms when given in a minute dose. Or, as he put it, "Let Likes Be Cured By Likes." He called this new science "homeopathy," from "homoios" (like) and "pathos" (suffering). Thus, practitioners of homeopathy were called "homeopaths." The practitioners of bloodletting and polypharmacy came to be called "allopaths" because their medical system was based not on like curing like but on medicines which had "allo" (different or opposite) actions. Over the next six years of his life, Hahnemann studied and experimented until he was sure he had discovered a scientific principle.

One of these early cases told Hahnemann that the remedies would be of use in epidemics. He had given a little girl Belladonna because of an inflammation of her finger joints. When a scarlet fever epidemic broke out, she was the only person in her family not to become ill. It was later proved that Belladonna was an important remedy in treating scarlet fever.

Hahnemann knew that others had taught "like is cured by like"; among them Paracelsus, and later Stahl of Denmark and Halle of Switzerland. However, Hahnemann was the first physician who developed this principle and turned it into a science.

Hahnemann had taken cinchona and developed the fever symptoms that cinchona cured; he had taken mercury and experienced the same symptoms mercury helped. His painter friend had ingested sepia off the brush and was cured by taking a homeopathic preparation of sepia. His findings had been validated and reproduced. But, he was not sure if the remedy could cure someone with those symptoms who had not ingested the same substance earlier. Would these substances cure an illness that came unexpectedly? He began to experiment and found that as long as the totality of the symptoms agreed—that is, most of the symptoms the person had fit the symptoms from taking the remedy in a crude dose—it would cure the illness.

Although Hahnemann was now certain of the principle of like curing like, he was still faced with the problem of finding the right dose for each particular illness. Remedies such as Veratrum Album, Belladonna, Aconitum Napellus and Lachesis were poisonous in too high a dose and, by the time they were diluted enough to be safe, they were ineffective.

Hahnemann began to experiment with different processes in order to make better remedies. In his day it was a common practice for alchemists to shake their preparations. Hahnemann tried this himself and discovered that if he shook, or succussed, the preparation, the beneficial properties were kept but the negative, or poisonous qualities, were erased. It was then possible to dilute a substance in order to make it safe, while still maintaining its curative properties.

In 1812, Hahnemann obtained a professorship at the University of Leipzig. He began to teach his theories and attracted a group of students who were willing to test the remedies on themselves. However, his denigration of orthodox medicine, his self-righteous attitude, and his affected way of dress made him a controversial figure at the school. He was sure he was right about homeopathy, yet the other professors saw his certainty as rigidity. Despite this, however, a small band of students gathered around him and began to investigate homeopathy.

They took minute doses of plant, animal, and mineral substances and kept careful records of the results. This process, which was called "pruefung" in German and in English became "proving," had strict rules to ensure that the results were as accurate as possible. The person testing a remedy did not know what he had taken; he had to be healthy; he had to eat a normal balanced diet so that whatever symptoms he developed could not be due to dietary changes; he could not smoke or drink alcohol. The person kept a careful record of how he felt; at the end these symptoms were compiled and other students tested to see if they developed the same symptoms after taking the same remedy. When people developed these same symptoms in the course of an illness, they were given the remedy, which most closely fit their case, and a record was kept of their improvement. By the end of Hahnemann's life, his followers had tested 600 remedies. These studies became a book called the *Materia Medica Pura*, which is still in print today.

The studies Hahnemann's students did were controversial, giving rise to arguments from physicians from the Brown, Brousais, or other schools of medicine. However, Hahnemann had credibility because early in his career he was known as a gifted chemist, researcher, and innovator.

Even before homeopathy, he was a proponent of gentle care for all patients, especially mental patients. He was given a chance to prove his medical theories about mental illness.

Known to be a proponent of compassionate care of the mentally ill, in 1792 Hahnemann was given a wing of Duke Ernst Von Sachsen-Gotha's castle as a private nursing home for mental cases. One of Hahnemann's violent patients was treated in a friendly manner, but all acts of violence were prohibited. His family visits were ended, and drugs were kept to a minimum. In seven months he went home, much improved, his violent episodes cured.

Despite his previous success in mental health, chemistry, and other fields, the progress of homeopathy did not run smoothly. There were several major incidents in Hahnemann's life that impeded the course of the new science.

Hahnemann treated two patients who at first prospered under his care and then relapsed when treated by allopaths or after sabotaging their own treatment. In 1792, the ailing duke Leopold asked Hahnemann to cure him, but he later relapsed. Some sources say he began to drink, others say he was treated by allopaths. Then he was asked to treat Prince Schwarzenberg of Austria, who had a stroke. He improved under Hahnemann's care, but was later bled by allopathic doctors and died. Since bloodletting was considered the preferred treatment and homeopathy was not, Hahnemann was indicted for the Prince's death. He was not held personally responsible, but for a time it was ruled that homeopathy was a secondary school of medicine and could only be practiced in rural areas where there were no allopaths readily available.

In addition, much of the controversy surrounding Hahnemann had to do with the way remedies were made. During a typhus epidemic spread by one of Napoleon's retreating armies, homeopathy was found to be much more effective than the traditional medicines the allopaths used. Perceiving homeopathy as a threat, the apothecaries sued Hahnemann over the right to make medicines. Because homeopathic remedies were made according to a precise process of dilution and succussion, Hahnemann and his followers insisted on making their own medicines. This enraged the apothecaries, who insisted on the right as a union to make all medicinal preparations. The homeopaths claimed that the apothecaries were not trained in making homeopathic remedies. Hahnemann appealed to the king, who had him treat one of his relatives, possibly Duke Leopold, as a test. As before, when the patient began to drink again, he relapsed. The king was then forced to side with the apothecaries. However, some apothecaries were persuaded to learn homeopathy as a result of the trial.

Over time, many physicians were eager to try homeopathy, but could not accept Hahnemann's concept of the infinitesimal dose. They could not believe such a small dose could have any effect.

A great deal of the controversy was based on the writings of Hahnemann himself. His foundational work, *The Organon of Natural Healing*, later called *The Organon of the Healing Art*, and his later work, the *Materia Medica Pura*, met with acclaim. However, his later work, *Chronic Diseases*, was criticized and misunderstood.

In *Chronic Diseases*, Hahnemann stated that seven-eighths of all diseases were caused by "psora" a hereditary taint. His detractors thought that what Hahnemann meant by "psora" was a later term for scabies, a common skin disease called "the itch." However, until 1890 psora included a broad range of ailments that included diseases of the glands and leprosy. This misunderstanding caused Hahnemann to be ridiculed, with detractors claiming that he thought all diseases stemmed from a minor skin disorder. However, in an effort to find the root cause of disease in an underlying process (called a "miasm") Hahnemann attempted to find a medical model of disease that answered the question of *why* we get sick.

Despite these battles, Hahnemann's theories were followed by many physicians; but sadly, he lived long enough to see his principles misused and distorted by individual practitioners. Hahnemann thought these "half-homeopaths" were worse than allopathic practitioners, because they distorted what he taught and then, when homeopathy failed to work, blamed the principles instead of their own applications.

After his wife, Henriette, died at the age of 67, he met the Marquise Marie Melanie d' Hervilly. Hahnemann was 79 and clearly taken by her; historical accounts vary as to whether she was sincere in her affection or ruthless in her possessiveness. Domestic life at the Hahnemann's mirrored the controversy of his professional life before eventual peace.

By some accounts, Melanie treated Hahnemann's children cruelly; in any case, she made a bad family situation worse. Hahnemann's son, Friedrich, had fallen from a horse and as a result was afflicted with a hunchback. A visible sign of his father's limitations as a doctor, he then incited Hahnemann's ire by marrying a widow with a child. Hahnemann accused him of not being worthy enough to find his own woman instead of marrying another man's wife. A physician in his own right, Friedrich did treat patients during epidemics and apparently was an accomplished musician, playing the piano on board to earn his ship's passage. But these gifts were not enough to impress Hahnemann, and he made Melanie his heir.

Melanie forced his daughters away from him, giving them their smaller inheritances but banishing them from his home. He had planned on enjoying a quiet retirement, but Melanie talked him into moving to Paris and opening a practice there.

Hahnemann practiced in Paris, with Melanie as his assistant, until he died at the age of 89, probably from pneumonia. Five years after he died, his coffin was moved and re-buried in Pere Lachaise cemetery where France's immortals rest; among Rossini, the poet Racine and playwright Moliere.

By the time Hahnemann died in 1843, almost the whole continent of Europe felt his influence. Homeopathy had spread to Russia, Mexico, Cuba, and the United States. It is fitting that Hahnemann's headstone reads *Non inutilis vixi*: "I have not lived in vain."

A Very Short (Well, *Short*, Anyway) History Lesson

It is beyond the scope of this book to discuss in detail a complete history of homeopathy in America. Nor is it necessary for someone to know the history to be able to practice homeopathy successfully for colds and flu. However, since people will be sure to ask questions about why homeopathy is not more prevalent in America today, a short (as short as I can make it, anyway) history lesson is in order. If you, (or someone in your family) are presently ill, please feel free to skip this chapter until a more opportune time presents itself and go ahead to the next section, *Taking Care Of Business.*

Medicine in America relied on bloodletting, polypharmacy, and other heroic medical measures, as did European medicine in Hahnemann's day. Bloodletting's major proponents who influenced American medicine were William Cullen and Benjamin Rush. Cullen, a Scotsman, had formulated convincing theories. He had categorized the actions of fever and thought a fever's progression was due to a spasm of the blood vessels. He said that bloodletting stopped these spasms and relieved the fever.

Benjamin Rush was more extreme in his views. He held that physicians should remove up to four-fifths of the blood supply in order to cure illness. He also maintained that it was harmful to the patient to stop the flow of blood once it began. Rush's influence led physicians to routinely remove between two to sixteen ounces of blood in the course of an illness.

Cutting veins was the most common form of bloodletting, but physicians also used cupping, blistering, purging, and sweating. Cupping was performed by placing a heated cup over the skin to bring the blood supply to the surface, where the veins were lanced. Blistering with irons caused second degree burns in order to provide an exit for fluids believed to cause the disease. Tarter Emetic, castor oil, magnesium, or calomel (a preparation of

Mercurius chloride) were given to cause vomiting, sweating, or emptying of the bowels.

One particularly nasty form of treatment to release bodily fluids was the seton. A shallow incision was made and either dried peas or a spool of cotton cord placed in the wound to absorb the discharge. As the surface layers of the spool were covered in pus, the thread was unrolled and cut off.

All of these treatments were used for any type of illness: fever, infections, colds, flu, arthritis, cancer. The treatment arsenal was very narrow. It's no wonder than the public was hungry for a better way to treat illness. Several alternative methods of treatment arose, paving the way for homeopathy.

The most popular of these was Thomsonianism. Thomsonianism was not based on the same principles as homeopathy. However, it was the first widespread medical system that gave responsibility for health back to the people. Thomsonianism empowered them to make their own choices.

Samuel Thomson was a country boy who dreamed of becoming a doctor. Unable to have formal schooling because of the expense, he learned herb lore from a neighborhood woman who prescribed for the sick. He began to treat his family and friends with herbs, and met with success.

Thomson believed in the underlying mythology of the Humoral Theory, which held that illness was a matter of imbalance between the four elements in the body: earth, air, fire, and water. He followed his herb concoctions with tonics or steam baths to cleanse the body.

Although Thomson's enemies tried to stop his practice after one of his patients died, the trial was a fiasco; it was proved that the preparations were harmless and he was cleared.

In 1813 he obtained patents for his treatments. For a fee, housewives could obtain a kit containing Thomsonian herbs, each box with a certificate proclaiming the owner a Thomsonian practitioner. The assumption was that they would treat only their own families, but most of them treated outsiders as well. There were few physicians on the frontier and the practitioners—mostly women—could not stand by and see others suffer. Women were relieved to spare their children the harsh methods of allopathic medicine, but in the process became unofficial medical practitioners.

As a result of the success of Thomsonianism, more and more people began to realize there could be an alternative treatment to bloodletting and polypharmacy.

◈ ◈ ◈ ◈ ◈

Two physicians, Hans Burch Gram and Henry Detwiller, were the first to bring homeopathy to America. Gram was a Dane born in Boston; Detwiller was German-Swiss. The Wesselhoft brothers, who practiced in Pennsylvania and Boston, joined them. Homeopathy on the East Coast met fertile ground. Many people who had been impressed with Thomsonian herb medicine were eager to try homeopathy.

However, the true father of homeopathy in America was not Hans Gram or Henry Detwiller, but a former allopath, Constantine Herring. Herring was asked by his superior, Dr. Robbie, to write a book defaming homeopathy for a publisher. Robbie had initially agreed to do it, but turned the project over to Herring when he did not have the time. After research, Herring became an adherent of homeopathy. He went on to found Homeopathic Medical College in Pennsylvania, which later became Hahnemann Medical College in Philadelphia.

James Tyler Kent, who began his career as an eclectic practitioner, continued Herring's work drawing from various medical theories at will. Later on in his career, he became a homeopath who trained a whole generation in the correct principles used by Hahnemann. He was professor of Materia Medica at the Homeopathic Medical College of St. Louis in the late 1800's. He developed the first repertory, containing 1,500 pages of symptoms and listing remedies associated with each one. The remedies are graded as to having a strong, moderate, and slight degree of correlation for each symptom.

Also worthy of honorable mention is Edward Bach. Born in 1886, he discovered the healing flower remedies and categorized them using emotional symptoms. He said that there were seven principal diseases of mankind: pride, cruelty, hate, self-love (selfishness), ignorance, instability, and greed. Each Bach Flower remedy treats emotional symptoms such as grief, resentment, or sadness. You can still buy Bach's flower remedies at most large health food stores.

Herring, Kent, and Bach all spent their lives in healing and the promotion of homeopathy as a valid method of cure. But it was the epidemics of the 1800's that boosted homeopathy into a recognized medical alternative in the United States. Cholera, diphtheria, measles, and yellow fever were rampant at this time and only homeopathy could defeat them.

After each epidemic, survivors, city officials, and medical personnel compared the allopathic and homeopathic treatment modes and homeopathy was the front-runner. When treating cholera, the allopathic death rate was 50% or usually higher, while homeopathy's death rate was 30% or usually lower. During the cholera epidemic in London in 1854, the London Homeopathic Hospital had a 16.4% death rate, the allopathic hospital 51.8%. Other sources say that for this same epidemic the death rates were 3% to 25% and between 50% to 60% respectively. During a Cincinnati outbreak in 1849, the homeopaths had a 3% death rate, versus up to a 70% death rate when using conventional allopathic means. Other sources cite similar statistics.

For these reasons homeopathy soon became the preferred type of treatment for people with money and the time to seek out a homeopath. Dana Ullman notes that homeopathy was patronized and championed by the elite. Mark Twain, William James, Louisa May Alcott, Harriet Beecher Stowe, and Henry Wadsworth Longfellow all were homeopathy clients. Homeopathy seemed to be a little stronger in the North, and Dana Ullman speculates that it was because abolitionists Zabina Eastman and William Lloyd Garrison were homeopathy supporters.

Depending on the area of the country, only one out of every three or four doctors was a homeopath, so finding one took a little dedication. Other sources estimate that between fifteen to thirty percent of all physicians were homeopaths. And, since homeopathic medical schools were the first to admit women, most of the early women doctors were probably homeopaths.

Dana Ullman reports that at the height of homeopathy in this country, there were twenty-two homeopathic medical schools; over 100 homeopathic hospitals; and over one thousand pharmacies.

It is hard to believe that homeopathy was once so popular in a culture that, today, barely knows what it is. In the next chapter, we shall see *why* that is, and why homeopathic relief for your colds and flu has been so hidden for the last several generations.

If Homeopathy Is So Great, Why Don't We Practice More Of It Today?

In the last chapter, you read about homeopathy and how it became a popular mode of cure. However, homeopathy's rise was not peaceful or quiet. From the time homeopathy came to America, the medical controversies surrounding it (and other forms of alternative medicine) threatened and changed Hahnemann's science. Impediments included persecution from doctors who followed other disciplines, the exact pharmaceutical practices in making remedies, the changes forced by the apothecaries' union, and Hahnemann's flamboyant and opinionated style all affected the growth of homeopathy. These controversies are why homeopathy went "underground" until its resurgence in the 1960's, 1970's, and 1980's.

One of the earliest controversies had to do with medical licensure. In the middle 1800's, even though medical school was out of the financial reach of many people, it was still not a quality education. Medical schools competed with one another for applicants, because they needed the cash. Often they took applicants who could barely read or write. While it was also possible to apprentice yourself to another doctor for training, that too was expensive and all too often the apprentice was a servant rather than a student. When the Thomsonians were accused of having poor training, they pointed out the sad state of medical education in general and asked for some kind of licensure, both to protect themselves and to ensure quality in the medical profession as a whole. It was the Thomsonians who called into question the four-month course that previously made up allopathic medical education.

Out of this criticism the American Medical Association (AMA) was formed in 1846. It was started ostensibly to improve the quality of medical education, but in reality to combat unorthodox methods of treatment, such as Chiropractic, Osteopathy, and Thomsonianism. For example, although one of their stated goals was to elevate the quality of medical education and practice, they preferred to do so by attacking other medical disciplines rather than by focusing on the reform of medical education within their own group.

In 1855 the AMA instituted the consultation clause, which stated that one could not be a member of the AMA and practice homeopathy or consult with a homeopath. Because AMA membership came with advantages like insurance and scholarship aid, and because the AMA was involved in medical licensure, there were many benefits to AMA membership. Because the medical license came not from the state government but from the local medical board, many physicians were afraid to practice without the AMA's endorsement.

The consultation clause became so ridiculous that one physician was suspended for consulting with a homeopath who happened to be his wife. Another physician was suspended for buying a product at a homeopathic pharmacy.

The entire Massachusetts Medical Society was accused of having homeopathic members and was denied a delegate at the AMA National Convention. Proponents of the Consultation Clause cited the homeopathic physicians for adhering to an "exclusive theory or dogma" that would preclude their membership.

But, perhaps the biggest problem with the consultation clause was over the signing of diplomas. Because there were homeopathic professors at the medical schools, and each professor of a subject signed the student's diploma, it was charged that those students should not be able to join the AMA because their diplomas had been signed by a homeopath; therefore, they had "consulted" with one.

The public, witnessing the controversy, had no sympathy for the doctors involved. Physicians in general lost credibility because the public regarded these squabbles as ridiculous. All people wanted was safe and effective treatment, regardless of what school or "dogma" the physician adhered to.

These controversies were fed by homeopathy's main detractor, Oliver Wendell Holmes, who said that the cures of homeopathy were only apparent cures and that the statistics proving homeopathy worked were unreliable. Dr. A. H. Okie said Holmes could not be correct, because homeopathy works on babies and animals who are immune to suggestion. He reminded

Holmes—and the public—that there were many medical theories that were once believed and later found out to be erroneous.

The next move from the AMA was to charge that the homeopathic medical schools were not as good as the allopathic ones. This criticism was unfounded, because homeopaths often attended the same schools as allopaths. They commissioned a study, the Flexner Report, to evaluate all medical schools and report on their quality.

The Flexner Report, issued in 1910, was negative about homeopathic education for the following reasons. First of all, they gave a lower grade to the homeopathic colleges because professors treated patients as well as taught classes. Secondly, they did not give credit for the courses in homeopathic *materia medica*, which meant that the homeopathy colleges appeared to require fewer courses. These apparent weaknesses made it look like the homeopaths had an inferior education.

After publication the Flexner Report was hotly debated, with detractors saying that the criterion was unfair and criticizing Flexner himself for not being a physician and, therefore, unable to judge the ideal medical education.

Another factor in weakening the homeopathic front was the death of heroic medicine. Between 1866 and 1870 bloodletting had come under attack by Dr. Thomas McGraw. After 1870 it was only used rarely for inflammation or cardiac congestion, and no longer taught in medical school. Now that heroic medicine was at an end, many critics of homeopathy, like H. C. Wood, said that homeopathy flourished only because it was safer than the harsh practices that preceded it.

When allopathic medicine became safer, many homeopaths began to see things of worth in that sort of medicine and adopted certain techniques for their own use. With the death of heroic medicine, the end of bloodletting, purging, blistering, and the decline of calomel, many homeopaths became eclectics, adopting ether for anesthesia and morphine for pain. Homeopaths began to increase dosages of remedies to be more in line with allopathic prescribers. They wanted to re-examine the law of similars and the infinitesimal dose. As a result, more natural substances were adopted.

At the same time, one of the basic tenets of homeopathy, that of the unknowability of the disease process, seemed threatened with the advent of the microscope. It was beginning to appear that the cause of all illness might someday become visible and be explained in physical terms.

The homeopaths were unable to provide a united front to fight these changes because, unfortunately, they were fighting among themselves about other issues. Homeopathy, like any movement, was not immune to factions. These factions proved deadly as the homeopaths were not able to collaborate and adjust to these social changes. They disagreed about how homeopathy should be practiced and the theories on which it was based.

Toward the end of the nineteenth century, the English homeopath Richard Hughes questioned the use of mental symptoms in determining the right remedy. Traditional homeopaths had long believed that fright, fear, excessive joy, and even unrequited love could affect the vital force, and that these symptoms could be used to find the right remedy in chronic illness. Hughes said that mental symptoms were not helpful in choosing a remedy; he used only low potencies to treat illness.

The opposite school was led by James Tyler Kent, the same practitioner discussed in the earlier chapter. Kent's lectures helped bring homeopathy back to its original practices. Kent managed to educate a generation of homeopaths away from frequent doses, exclusive use of low potencies, and mixing remedies. Today, when the description "classical homeopathy" is applied to a practice, it signifies a practitioner who practices as Hahnemann taught homeopathy, a legacy that was preserved by Kent's work.

Homeopaths were also divided about the use of very high potencies—called "infinitesimals." Still others were divided about Hahnemann's theory of miasms as being the underlying cause of illness. Still others were fighting about the status and efficacy of eclectics who used several different systems on the same patient.

There was too much disagreement among homeopaths. Kent's consolidating work was unable to settle the issues in time for the homeopaths to fight the real threat to their existence: the allopathic school of medicine that did not follow the law of similars and the rules of dilution and succussion that made homeopathy work.

The other weakness in the homeopathic system is that it was, and is still, not a lucrative way of practicing medicine. Homeopathy has always demanded more time from the physician in order to treat the patient. The income of any allopathic physician is almost always greater than that of any homeopath, because the allopath is able to see more patients in the same amount of time. This disparity could hardly be attractive to a new physician, who was anxious to start practicing and earning a substantial income.

Another factor in the decline of homeopathy was the belief that neither school, the allopaths nor the homeopaths, had the whole truth. The pure homeopaths, or "Hahnemannians" as they were called, appeared rigid for adhering to the old principles. Allopaths were looked upon as uncompromising and dedicated to protecting their turf at the expense of better treatment for the patient. The eclectics thought they had the best of both systems and even put out a paper called *The Medical Union* in an effort to heal the breach. There was a movement toward a search for the truth rather than adherence to a particular dogma or set of theories.

After the turn of the century, in the spirit of "If you can't beat 'em, join 'em," and after years of bitter fighting, the AMA grandfathered in all homeopaths. All practicing homeopaths were absorbed into the AMA and their original practices changed and eroded. Homeopaths began to use high dose undiluted remedies and dropped the tenet of "like cures like." Their practice was contaminated by principles of allopathic medicine, and since homeopathy will not work unless the principles are followed, it looked like homeopathy was at an end.

◈ ◈ ◈ ◈ ◈

Homeopathy has left its mark on medicine forever. Because of homeopathy the use of bloodletting, purging, calomel, tartar emetic, and other inhumane practices were discontinued: Polypharmacy diminished, most doctors believing that there was a synergistic effect of drugs, and the fewer, the better. Homeopathy was the forerunner of desensitizing allergy treatment, and gave the medical field nitroglycerine for heart disease. In short, Homeopathy left a belief in medical treatment that *less* was *better* while alerting physicians to new and safer medications.

These changes wrought by homeopathy were deep. They made it seem as though homeopathy was meant to shape medicine, but not endure as its own discipline and mode of treatment.

However, Hahnemann's system of medicine was down, but not out. The last thirty or forty years have seen a resurgence of homeopathy in this country. Let's look at some of the reasons for a renewed interest in homeopathy in the next chapter.

Down But Not Out:
The "Return" Of Homeopathy

Homeopathy may have been driven underground in the United States in the earlier part of this century, but it is important to remember homeopathy still flourished in most other countries. England, India, Mexico, Europe, Australia, Russia, Central and Latin America, and Sweden all made homeopathy a common alternative to allopathic medicine for many generations.

Dana Ullman says in his book *Homeopathic Medicine For Children and Infants*:

> . . .England's Royal Family has been under homeopathic care since the 1830's. . . . organized medicine in Europe has not been as antagonistic to homeopathy as American medical organizations have been. . .One third of the French population uses homeopathic medicines, and 32 percent of French family physicians prescribe them. One-fifth of all German physicians use homeopathic medicines; 42 percent of British physicians refer patients to homeopathic physicians, and 45 percent of Dutch physicians consider homeopathic medicines effective. . . . according to a recent market research survey by London's Frost and Sullivan, Ltd., the field of alternative and complementary medicine, including homeopathy, is expanding so quickly that it was Europe's second biggest growth industry during the 1980's, second only to the computer industry.[1]

---

[1]Dana Ullman, *Homeopathic Medicine For Children and Infants* (New York: Jeremy P. Tarcher, 1992), pp. xvii-xviii.

Since almost every other country allowed homeopathy to flourish, it seems a misnomer to say that homeopathy made a "return." It may be more proper to say that America "rediscovered" homeopathy in the 60's and its popularity has grown ever since.

Reasons for a return to homeopathy are as individual as the people reading this book, but I'll list some general points:

1. There's been a disenchantment with traditional medical treatment, especially drug treatment. Americans are becoming aware that treatment with drugs often comes at a price. Thalidomide served as a wake-up call, but we have all experienced our own prescription side effects: addictions to antihistamines or tranquilizers; diarrhea and candida from antibiotics; heart disease from Phen-fen. Reports of iatrogenic, or treatment-induced, illnesses are only as far away as the evening news. Like those Thomsonian housewives, we are still looking for safe and effective means of treatment. Often, allopathic medicine will not give us that option.

2. A second reason is the resentment over rising medical costs. It is astonishing to me that insurance companies are not more eager to cover alternative medicine as a measure to cut costs. Since homeopathy is extremely inexpensive, even for people who are uninsured, it has become a good treatment of choice for people for whom medical care must be on a cash-and-carry basis. Homeopathic self-care costs the time to train practitioners and clients and very little money. In most cases, a visit to a homeopathic practitioner is cheaper than a visit to an M.D. or D.O.

3. More people want to take responsibility for their own care. Previous generations were willing to have all their medical decisions made by the physician. Now, there is a wish to be more involved in one's own care. Because a careful reporting of symptoms is essential to the case, homeopathy certainly fills this need.

4. People are tired of impersonal care. Most homeopathic practitioners spend more time on a case; therefore, there is not the "quick in and out the door" of other doctor's visits.

In all fairness, much of the pressure to see a lot of clients in a small amount of time is not the physician's fault. Some physicians may be motivated by greed, but most are faced with expensive malpractice insurance costs, rent, supply costs, staff salaries, and repayment of student loans, while fighting to make a living threatened by HMO's and PPO's. All this means that they must be ruthless with their time in order to survive. It's no wonder that this is often perceived by the patient as cold and impersonal treatment. But no matter the cause, this experience has done a lot to make people seek alternative medicine.

And, finally:

5. The inadequacy of allopathic medical treatment for some disorders has led many people to alternative medicine. Not only are people disenchanted with what doctors are prescribing, there are instances where allopathic treatment has not been successful for their particular illness. Treatment for asthma, fibromyalgia, arthritis, lupus, allergies, and yes—colds and flu—are often unsuccessful and lead clients into alternative treatment.

◈ ◈ ◈ ◈ ◈

So large has the practice of homeopathy grown that today there are between 2,000 homeopathic medical doctors and osteopaths; 750 to 1,000 natural physicians who practice homeopathy, at least 500 veterinarians, and 300 to 500 dentists. In addition, several thousand chiropractors practice some form of homeopathy. Not to mention the hundreds of humble lay homeopaths, of which I am one.

No matter what your reasons are for investigating homeopathy, you're in good, and numerous, company. In the next chapter, you will see that your curiosity is well founded, and that there is evidence that homeopathy is a valid medical process for you to treat your own colds and flu.

How Do I Know
This Is Going To Work?

When Hahnemann gave a remedy to his students, his system for giving a remedy and watching the results was called "Pruefung" which is German for "test." Because "pruefung" sounds like the English word "proving", that is what English speaking homeopaths call this process, as if the test *proved* the remedies work, which in a way they do. Hahnemann's testing of remedies on individuals was the first truly scientific medicine, based on scientific principles of observation and repetition.

Physicians of his day often said that the remedies only worked because people expected them to work. This is called the *placebo effect*. Although the placebo effect can be a powerful one, and it is true that ineffective drugs can cure because of this effect, this cannot be true of homeopathy. The remedies have been shown to work on infants, animals, and comatose people, where the placebo effect would not be operative.

In the late 1800's, life insurance companies gave lower rates to those who went to homeopathic physicians, because they lived longer. Larger sums were paid for homeopathic patients when they died than allopathic ones.

There are other indications that homeopathy works. Among them is the Chaos theory, which has shown us that minute changes can eventually lead to huge differences. Even a small change can have an avalanche effect.

Another strong proof for homeopathy is the Biphasic Principle of Pharmacy. This law was initially discovered by two researchers, Hugo Schulz, a scientist, and Rudolf Arndt, a psychiatrist. It was originally called the Arndt-Schulz law.

It would be logical to suppose that if a drug in a maximum dose heals a condition, then as the drug is decreased, it will reach a level where it will be too weak to have an effect on the organism at all. Finally, in a minute dose it will be to weak for the organism to perceive and use it. This would be a logical way of looking at medication.

However, the Biphasic Principle states that, to the contrary, drugs have increased effects in a large dose, and as the amount of a drug decreases these effects will get smaller. Then there comes a time when a very small dose will have the *opposite* effect of a larger dose.

Put in another way, it states that strong doses *halt* a physiological activity, medium doses *inhibit* the same physiological activity, and weak doses *stimulate* the same physiological activity. This law, also called "Hormesis" was verified in the 1920's. It shows that even the minute doses of homeopathic remedies will have an effect.

There have been many studies that have verified the efficacy of a minimum dose. One of the most famous was that of W. E. Boyd. From 1941-42, Boyd studied the results of minute doses of mercurius chloride on seed germination and discovered an infinitesimal dose to have an effect.

There have been many studies showing the efficacy of homeopathy for colds and flu. In 1991, three professors of medicine from the Netherlands published in the *British Medical Journal* the results of a 25-year study of respiratory infections, hay fever, and other illnesses treated with homeopathy. Twice as many people got over the flu in 48 hours if they took Oscillococcinum (Anas Barbarae) than those who did not. Similar studies have shown that while combination remedies have proved effective against flu, single remedies have proved better.

Livingston, in *Homeopathy*, November 1970, published an earlier influenza study. One group was given a homeopathic flu remedy and another not. Those who were not treated homeopathically lost eight and one-half times the workdays than those who were treated. Fewer became ill and if they did get ill, they missed less work time.

Several more recent studies have shown the efficacy of homeopathy, and there have even been "studies of the studies" in an effort to explore its cure rates.

Homeopathy is popular enough for the Dutch Ministry of Welfare, Public Health, and Cultural Affairs to finance a study of the research showing the efficacy of homeopathy. Jos Kleijnen, Paul Knipschild, and Gerben ter Riet state that although they thought at first homeopathy was "implausible," by the end of the study they found "The amount of positive evidence even among the best studies came as a surprise to us."[2]

They came to this conclusion after examining material from computer searches, articles in clinical research, textbooks, and journals of homeopathy. They also visited manufacturers of homeopathic remedies. After more than three years of research, they assigned point scores for these studies points based on how well they were conducted. Their criteria included: whether or not the patients symptoms were adequately described, if the sample was truly random or not, if the intervenon was well described, the quality of the double bind study, the effectiveness of the study's measurements, and if the results published could be checked by the reader. When they looked at all the available literature, they found 16 trials that had gathered points of 60 or more that seemed the most reliable.

Remedies tested included Oscillococcinum, Arnica Montana, Gelsemium, Eupatorium Perfoliatum, Pulsatilla, Aconite, Bryonia, Phosphorus, and combination remedies.

These studies concluded that homeopathy works. Out of 105 trials, 81 indicated positive results with 24 indicating no positive results.

In a similar later study, Klaus Linde, Nicole Clausius, Gilbert Ramirez, Dieter Melchart, Florian Eitel, Larry V. Hedges, and Wayne B. Jonas examined available data and found that, when weighted considering the bias of the researchers, homeopathy came out even more effective. In their study, 95% of the previous research showed homeopathy as being more effective.

It is beyond the scope of this book to explore the laboratory evidence supporting homeopathy. Readers who seek more information are referred to Dana Ullman's chapter on research in *The Consumer's Guide to Homeopathy*; and G. Ruthven Mitchell's book, *Homeopathy*, which contains an in-depth study of the 1970 influenza experiment cited above. For those of you ready for a more scholarly approach, see the chapters on cell, human, and

---

[2]Jos Kleijnen, Paul Knipschild, and Gerben ter Riet, "Clinical Trials Of Homeopathy," *British Medical Journal*, (9 February 1991, vol. 302), pp. 316-323.

animal studies in Paulo Bellavite and Andrea Signorini's *Homeopathy: A Frontier In Medical Science.*

All right, now that you are aware of evidence that shows the efficacy of homeopathy, are you ready to look at some differences between allopathy and homeopathy? On we go. . .

What's the Difference Between Homeopathic and Allopathic Medicine?

We are all called on to learn to make changes in our lives. As growing and developing infants we had to learn to focus our eyes, and later to eat with a spoon, crawl and then walk. We learned to talk, and by the end of kindergarten most of us knew our colors and beginning numbers, and many of us learned to write our names. Then later we had to learn the tools and techniques of grooming, academic study, managing our careers, our personal finances, adjusting to living with first a spouse and then, perhaps, children. Later in life, we had to change again after the death of a parent or a spouse, learn to handle our retirement time and how to live on a fixed income. It starts at birth and goes on until we die—and who's to say that there is not some change after death as well?

There are many differences between homeopathy and allopathic medicine. Those who want to practice homeopathy, even on themselves or their families, need to learn new concepts and make some fundamental changes in how they view illness and how it should be treated. Learning these fundamental rules is not difficult. If you read through this chapter and remember these principles when you treat yourself or your family with homeopathic remedies, you will do well.

One of the problems in writing this section is that there is no good word for non-homeopathic physicians. I hate to use the term "traditional" since homeopathy has existed for hundreds of years. "Orthodoxy" doesn't seem to work, either, because it implies homeopaths are non-orthodox, and seems to betray their years of experimental verification. I really prefer the term "allopath", meaning a physician who tends to treat with drugs that produce a different, or opposite, effect than the symptom. This is a term most homeopaths agree on, since "homeopath" defines them as treating with a like substance.

So now, to begin; here are the differences between homeopathy and allopathic medicine:

1. Homeopaths believe in the vital force, which is the force that animates the body and keeps it well. This force is called "chi" in acupuncture. The goal of homeopathic treatment is to strengthen the vital force in order for the body to fight illness. Although physicians are free to believe in a force, usually called "the will to live," this idea is not a foundational tenet of allopathic medical care.

2. Although theoretically they know better, allopaths treat conditions as though they believe that the symptoms of an illness come from the illness itself. For example, the nasal discharge is caused by the virus causing the cold. The fever is caused by the infection that prompts it.

Homeopaths believe that symptoms are the body's attempt to heal itself. The nasal discharge is an effort to clear the mucus membranes of the offending pollen or virus; the fever is the body's attempt to kill the invading virus. Homeopathy seeks to work with the body to help the body's defenses heal the illness and restore health.

3. Homeopaths believe in Herring's Law Of Cure, which was a principle taught in all medical schools a hundred years ago. It states that cure proceeds from above downward, from within outward, from the most important organs to the least important organs, and in the reverse order of the symptoms. This means that when a person is treated, the illness first heals from the top of the head and moves toward the feet, the most important organs heal first, the healing process moves from within outward, and the most recent symptoms will heal up first.

In a practical sense, this means that when you treat a cold or flu, the most recent symptom is the first to heal. Let's say you caught a cold that progressed this way:

Monday: Stuffy nose
Tuesday: Stuffy nose, scratchy throat
Wednesday: Stuffy nose, scratchy throat, ear pain and headache

When you take a remedy, the headache and ear pain probably will be the first to get better, followed by the throat pain and the stuffy nose.

Sometimes it's easier to see Herring's Law of cure go from the top down. Often, the first sign is a return of energy, a feeling of renewed interest in life. These are mental symptoms that also follow Herring's law of cure, because mental processes are much more important to your survival than your nose.

Most homeopaths believe in this theory and use it to assess how the cure is progressing. Allopathic physicians, however, are unfamiliar with this law and do not use it as a means of understanding the disease or curative processes.

4. Homeopaths believe that everyone inherits a disease process. This process grows and changes throughout our lives, depending on what physical and emotional stresses we have, losses we incur, nutritional choices we make, toxic elements we are exposed to, and other factors. Allopathic physicians tend to see illness as an event in the life of an organism, the cause of which is either external, in the case of a cold, or a problem with the functioning of the body, the chemistry gone awry.

Homeopathic physicians tend to see illness as part of an ongoing process that they are trying to stop and "roll back" to an earlier era in the life of the organism when the patient was healthier. Allopathic physicians tend to see illness, especially acute illness, as an isolated event, an exposure to an invader from outside.

5. Homeopaths believe that illness is an unseen, dynamic force with an unseen, dynamic cure. Allopaths believe that illness has a physical cause and therefore, a physical cure.

Allopaths tend to believe that all illness has a scientific cause, which can be measured; if we haven't measured it yet, it just means our technology is not sophisticated enough, not that it *can't* be measured. For example, we may not know how aspirin works, but it must work on some cellular level, which we cannot yet measure.

Homeopaths believe that the true cause of illness is unseen and dynamic, and therefore requires the unseen, dynamic force of a homeopathic remedy to cure it.

This is why the minute doses of homeopathic remedies do not pose a problem for the homeopath. He knows that the energy within the remedies is invisible, but that does not mean it is not there or that it will not be effective.

This reliance on a minute dose is what sets homeopathy apart from herbalism. Herbal doses are still too crude to act on the vital force of the body and tend to act in ways similar to allopathic drugs. Although herbal medicine can be safer than drug therapy, and as effective, it does not work in the same way as homeopathy.

6. Homeopaths believe that the lower the dose and the less frequently you dose a person, the better. Allopaths, when met with failure, will strengthen the dose to increase the medication, or change the medication.

Homeopaths believe that the fewer doses and the lower the strength of the remedy, the better. They do not want to repeat doses too frequently, not wanting to interfere with the vital force of the body that is seeking to make that person well. They see their role as supportive of the body's natural processes.

Allopathic traditional medicine is usually more aggressive in treating illness; they tend to see their role as more invasive.

7. Homeopaths believe in *Similia Similibus Curentur*, "Let likes be cured by likes": that is, a disease can be cured by minute doses of the same substance that would cause these symptoms in a crude dose.

For example, a crude dose of digitalis would give you the same heart palpitations and pain that a minute dose of digitalis would cure. In this same way, belladonna when ingested in a crude form would give you the same violent carotid pounding, dilated pupils, and red face that it cures in a minute dose.

Homeopaths have treated lead or mercury poisoning by giving minute potencies of mercury or lead. It seems to clean out the body of these residues.

Allopathic medicine has always worked by giving people a drug that will give the opposite effect. For example, if you have excess stomach acid, an allopathic physician will usually give you a base that will cut the stomach acid. If you have a runny nose, you will take something to dry up your nose.

8. Homeopaths treat the whole person, realizing that one body system cannot be separated from another. They look at mental and emotional symptoms, even when treating a cold. Allopathic physicians tend to tread a body part as though it's isolated. If they perceive mental symptoms, say, associated with trauma, they will treat them, but for garden-variety colds and flu, mental symptoms are not treated and are not used to find the right

medication. Homeopaths realize that each person is a whole being and must be looked at as a whole.

9. Similar to the above is the homeopathic belief that each person is a unique individual who has his own individual disease process and way of healing. If you have a head cold, no one in the world has ever had the same head cold as you This is why you require individual treatment, and this is why ten people with head colds will require ten different remedies. No one will ever be ill in the same way as you are. Therefore, each person needs to be approached on an individual basis.

10. It is typical for allopathic physicians to treat all people who have the same illness the some way. Sometimes this is described as a "disease entity," that is, a disease can be separated from the person. Allopathic physicians usually start treatment with a preferred drug and then go on to the next medication if the previous one doesn't work. Rarely do they tailor treatment to the individual unless the first choice of medication doesn't work. Homeopaths treat each person by giving him the remedy that fits his particular case. For example, five different asthma patients may require five different remedies.

11. Allopaths tend to believe that drugs only act on one part of the body. For example, they will give antihistamines to clear up a runny nose. They may know that these antihistamines usually will dry out the whole person's body, but they don't act as if it will or acknowledge it. If the person develops dry cracked lips as a result of taking the antihistamines, the physician will usually call it a "side effect" instead of acting as though the dry lips are a standard part of the drug's action.

Conversely, the homeopath will realize that the remedy will effect every part of the body: mental, emotional, and physical symptoms. It's not at all unusual for the temperament of a child to improve if he takes repeated doses of a remedy for a cold that happens to fit his mental as well as physical symptoms.

◈ ◈ ◈ ◈ ◈

Although the conceptual gulf between homeopathy and allopathy seems wide, many allopathic M.D.'s have changed their practices to become homeopathic M.D.'s. Surely it is not too difficult for us, even though we may have a lifetime of unlearning to do.

Now that you've read and (hopefully) understood these concepts, let's go on to learn how to treat our own colds and flu with homeopathy.

Part Two:

TAKING CARE OF BUSINESS

The Attorneys Made Me Put This In: Or, When To See A Physician For A Cold Or Flu

We've all heard the old joke about colds and flu: you're afraid you're going to die and also afraid you won't. The apex of a cold or flu can certainly feel miserable, and it's sometimes hard to know when to admit defeat and go to the doctor's office and when you can treat yourself.

What I always look for is if the cold or flu is going through some sort of progression. For example, is the tight chest turning into a wet cough as the fluid is being coughed up and expelled? Is the sore throat better and the stuffy nose turning into a runny one? These are the normal progressions of a cold, and when I see a change I at least feel that the cold is not "stuck" and not moving out. I am checking if the phlegm is lessening or discharging, if the fever is lower, if the periods of non-fever are lengthening, or if the quality of sleep is getting better.

But, as we all know, there are times when colds just don't seem to go *anywhere*. You feel like you are not getting better and you need professional advice.

Dr. Nina Cahan, a Dallas area OBGYN and pediatrician, details the following symptoms that mean the cold or flu is too severe for self-treatment.

If you do have any of the symptoms listed here, it **does not** mean that you can't use homeopathy as an adjunct treatment to help you get over your cold or flu. It just means that you should contact a licensed physician—a medical doctor or a doctor of osteopathy—in order to make sure that what you have is truly a cold or flu and obtain his diagnostic advice.

Symptoms that should be checked by a physician are:

1. Any fever or cold or flu when you are pregnant.
2. If you are over 65.
3. Excessive fatigue and weakness after a case of the flu, especially if you are loosing weight as well.
4. If you have emphysema or insulin dependent diabetes.
5. If you have asthma and the cold is making the asthma worse.
6. Flu that does not begin to get better in a week.
7. Flu that starts to get better but relapses.
8. If you are coughing up yellow phlegm.

And, most importantly:

9. **Anytime you feel like the cold or flu is out of your control and nothing is helping.**

Hot. . .Hotter. . .Burning Up. . . Or, When To See A Physician About A Fever

For some of us, of all the cold and flu symptoms, the most frightening is fever. Granted, the nasal discharge is annoying, and the coughing may be embarrassing or exhausting. But fever is by far the most frightening symptom of a cold or flu and probably the most debilitating.

For home care of a fever, the most important treatment is to drink plenty of fluids. Remember that your higher body temperature is burning up moisture, so if you ought to be drinking ten eight-oz. glasses of fluid daily. Even 12 or 14 glasses would not be too much when running a fever.

But when should you get medical care for a fever? Dr. Cahan says:

1. In infants under two months of age, *any* fever.
2. Older infants: more than 101°F rectal temperature.
3. Any child who has ever had a febrile seizure.
4. Anyone with a fever of 102°F or higher.
5. Anyone regardless of age who has extreme lethargy with fever.
6. Anyone with asthma that the fever makes worse.
7. Anyone with a fever who is not drinking some type of fluid.
8. Anyone with a fever who is not urinating at least two to three times a day.
9. Anyone with a fever whose eyes become sensitive to light.

10.   Anyone with fever accompanied with neck
         stiffness or severe headache.
11.   Anyone who is an insulin dependent diabetic.

Once again, meeting one of the above criteria and having to consult your physician does not mean that homeopathy will be of no use to you. Often, you may have one of these symptoms, call your doctor, and because the condition is viral, there may be no allopathic treatment for fever beyond cough syrup, acetaminophen or aspirin, fluids, and bed rest. In that case, homeopathy can be helpful in getting over the illness more quickly.

When should you go back to work or send a child back to school after a fever? I usually tell my clients to stay home until they have been without a fever for 24 hours, then return to their duties as gradually as possible.

How To Take Care Of Your Remedies

I often tell my clients that there are no errors in selecting a homeopathic remedy. Even if a remedy purchased does not work for that particular cold or flu, they need only tuck it away against some future time when it might be needed for another illness, for themselves or someone within the family or their circle of friends. All the remedies in this book, with the possible exception of Oscillococcinum and Influenzinum, can be used to treat a variety of ailments.

With proper handling homeopathic remedies will last indefinitely, as long as you follow a few simple rules:

1.   Keep the remedies away from direct sunlight.
2.   Recap tightly.
3.   Throw away any remedy that falls out. *Never* try to put remedies you have touched or spilled back into the bottle.
4.   If you have to transport the remedy you can wrap it in clean paper.
5.   Keep the remedies away from X-rays.
6.   Never, never, never put the remedies through the x-ray metal detector at the airport. If you must travel with remedies, put them in a plastic bag, hand them to one of the clerks and say, "This is medication that cannot be x-rayed." They will look at it and hand it back to you on the other side. If that doesn't work for you in these post 9-11 times, pack it in your checked bags if they are not to be x-rayed. Or, if you are allowed by airport authorities, keep it in your pocket; the metal detector you walk through will not hurt it.

7.   Keep the remedies away from strong smells, such
       as cleaning solutions, paint, and of course, the "big
       three": camphor, menthol, and eucalyptus.
8.   Never put your remedies on top of or within
       two feet of a television, computer, telephone,
       or any other electronic device.

Although remedies may be stamped with an expiration date, this is a legal requirement, not a practical one. Remedies don't go "bad" if they are handled correctly. If you follow these rules, your remedies should last indefinitely.

Twenty Questions To Ask About Colds and Flu (OK, So It's More Than Twenty. . .But Don't Despair. . .)

The first thing to remember when learning to take a cold case is that what you are trying to do is listen to the sick person describe his illness. Often, you are listening for what they *don't say* as well as for what they *say*.

For example, there is a great deal of difference between these three responses to the question "What do you feel like eating?"

Mom: What do you feel like eating?

Kid 1: Uh. . .I donno. . .maybe pizza or something. . .

Kid 2: Tacos! Can we have tacos? I want tacos! With plenty of hot sauce!

Kid 3: Ugh! Dinner already?

The first answer, the answer of someone who really doesn't care if the eats or not, is indifferent. Also, if pizza is a staple in your child's diet, you can't really count on wanting pizza as being a symptom of his current cold. However, if your child wants something he doesn't usually crave, that's a good clue. The second child has a marked preference for spicy food, and you might be able to use "craves spicy food" as a clue to finding the appropriate remedy. For the third answer you might safely mark "loss of appetite," because he has no wish for anything to eat.

With a little practice this is easy to spot; after all, you live in the same house, don't you? And as a parent, you can't help but notice your child's needs, wants, what is usual behavior for your child and what is not.

Taking a case is simpler than it looks, as long as you can listen and observe what your child, friend, or spouse is not saying. If the sick person is you, it's easy to apply these same observations to yourself.

◈ ◈ ◈ ◈ ◈

When you are looking for a remedy for a cold, you are looking for the remedy that fits the totality of the patient's symptoms. You will be looking for symptoms of the whole person, but in a restricted sense because you are only looking for symptoms that are likely in colds or flu. A homeopath seeking to help a long term or chronic disease process deals with a broader range of symptoms. Although it is possible that a chronic disease may become better as a result of homeopathic cold or flu prescription, your goal is to treat the flu. Therefore, you will look for symptoms of the cold or flu.

It's helpful if you do your search in logical order. Below are the questions you will want to keep in your mind when you narrow down your search for the correct remedy.

Please don't feel that you have to ask all of these questions of everyone to get the right remedy. What you might do is read them to yourself before you examine them, so that you have an idea of what you are looking for. A lot of the time, if you do ask a question, the answer will be no, sealing off that avenue and making your job shorter. This shortcut is ultimately less effective, because the patient may not then expound on other related symptoms. *What's important about these questions is that you know what you are looking for.*

The following questions are phrased in the third person, but you can just as easily apply them to yourself.

1. *What was he doing when the cold came on?* Had he been chilled, out in the wind, under some physical or emotional stress? Overworked? Had a major disappointment? Did he just suffer an injury or have surgery? Was there a change in the weather? Did he eat food that could have been tainted? In other words, do you feel anything unusual happened to him that could have made him susceptible to the cold or flu?

2. *How is his state of mind?* How are his memory and concentration? Is there a type of thinking he prefers? Conceptual, abstract? Is he artistic or mechanically minded? Is he unusually fearful, anxious, depressed, or angry? Is he afraid? If so, of what? How is his temper? Has he been startling easily? Has he been sad? If so, what time of day does he seem to be worse or better? There is a great temptation to blame emotional states on circumstance, such as, "Well, he has been sad, but his pet died, or his friend moved away. . ." You have to use your own judgment on how much

circumstance has to do with the patient's emotional state. I usually look for excessive patterns of thought—maybe the dog did die, but has he been crying overmuch? Yes, he is awaiting important test results—but is he anxious out of proportion to the event?

3. *Any head symptoms*? How does his head feel? Does he have vertigo (dizziness)? If so, what time of day does it happen? What makes the vertigo better? What makes it worse? Does he have a headache? If so, where does it hurt on his head? What does it feel like? What makes the headache better or worse? Is it worse at a certain time of day? Is his scalp sore?

4. *Is his face any different*? Is his face swollen, pale, red, and if so, is it on both sides equally? Does he have circles under his eyes? Does his face hurt? If so, where?

5. *Any eye symptoms*? Are they swollen, red, itchy, tearing? If they are tearing, do the tears burn? How do his eyes feel when they are moved and used? Are his pupils dilated? Are they sensitive to light? Are there any disturbances of vision, such as specks? When are the eyes better or worse? What makes them better or worse?

6. *How do his ears feel?* Does he have roaring or other sounds in his ears? Is he sensitive to noise? Are his ears hot or red? Is there pus in his ears? Does the ear pain travel down the neck or anywhere else? Does he feel like he has fluid in his ears?

7. *How does his nose feel?* Does he have a nasal discharge? How does the nasal discharge smell to him? What color (green, yellow, clear) is it? What consistency is it? (ropy, thick, thin, watery). Are both nostrils equally stuffy, running, or blocked? Does the discharge alternate between being runny and blocked? Does the discharge burn the nostrils or the upper lip? How does his nose feel? Is his nose sore? What color is the outside of his nose? Is he sneezing, and does the sneezing relieve his stuffiness?

8. *How are his mouth and tongue*? Is his tongue coated? Does it have any cracks in it? Is it flabby, showing the imprint of the teeth? Does he have mouth ulcers? Are his mouth and tongue sore? Are his lips dry or cracked?

9. *Does he have a sore throat?* Is his throat red, white, swollen? Does his throat feel constricted? Is it worse swallowing, worse when he doesn't swallow, or is it sore all the time? *How* does it hurt? Scraped, tingling, raw? Any sensation of a lump,

splinter, or hair in his throat? How much does it hurt? Are the throat muscles so constricted that liquids come out of his nose?

10. *And his larynx?* Is he hoarse? Does it hurt in the larynx when he coughs or breathes in? Is he hoarse at a certain time of day? Is he more hoarse or less hoarse when he talks a while? Does he have mucus in his larynx? What does his voice sound like?

11. *Ask about his neck and back.* Are they painful or stiff? If so, where? What kind of neck or back pain does he have? Throbbing, aching, etc.? What makes the pain better or worse? Does he feel like the muscles of his back are sore, or does it feel like it's the bones that are aching? Are his lymph nodes swollen?

12. *Any chest symptoms?* How well is he breathing? Is he short of breath? Is his chest burning or constricted? Does he have any chest pain?

13. *Is he coughing?* If so, is it dry, wet, hacking, painful in his chest or head? Is it worse or better lying down? When he coughs something up, what does it look like? Is there a time of day when the cough is worse or better? What makes the cough worse or better? Does the cough make him choke, retch, or vomit? Is he coughing up blood?

14. *Extremities?* How do his arms, legs, hands and feet feel? Are they cold or hot? Are they stiff or sore? Is he having any muscle cramps, numbness, or tingling? Do his arms or legs fall asleep easily?

15. *Does he have stomach trouble?* Does he have cramps, belching, nausea, or diarrhea? If he has cramps or nausea, is it worse after he eats or before he eats? What makes the cramps better or worse? Has he been vomiting? Does he have any appetite? If he has diarrhea, what is it like? (Watery, unusual color, etc.) Does the diarrhea burn? Does his stomach feel bloated or heavy?

16. *What about food?* Is he thirsty? What does he want to eat or drink? What does he definitely *not* want to eat or drink? What disagrees with him, gives him gas or stomach pains or diarrhea? Does his food taste unusual? (Please note: an *aggravation* is a stomach upset from eating a particular food. An *aversion* is an avoidance of a particular food; he doesn't want to eat it, but if he did, it wouldn't make him physically ill. Of course, you can have a food that you have both an aversion to which gives

you an aggravation. It is important to make the distinction when taking a case.)

17. *How is he sleeping?* Has he been restless, waking up in the night? If so, what time? Has he had any nightmares or dreams that he remembers? What position does he sleep in?

18. *Is he running a fever?* How high has it been? Does he have chills? How do the chills and fever come on? Is he perspiring, and if so, where?

19. *What makes him feel better?* Does he want to be left alone, have a hot bath, bundle up, be outdoors, have company, eat, not eat? What time of day does he feel better?

20. *What makes him feel worse?* Is he worse after he eats, after talking, after not sleeping, when he first gets up? Are there drinks or food that makes him feel worse? What time of day does he feel worse?

21. G*eneral questions?* Did the illness come on suddenly or gradually? Do the symptoms start in the chest and go up to the nose or vice versa? Do the symptoms alternate, such as the nasal discharge alternating with headache? Do they seem to be left or right sided, or move from right to left? Which side is worse? Are his senses dull or hyperacute? Does he have sensations like something blowing on him? Are there changes in behavior? Does he have any unusual postures? Coughing with his hand on his chest, sleeps sitting up? Do tight clothes bother him? Is he trembling or shaking? Do any of the pains shift from one part to another?

Use phrases such as "what else?" or "anything else?" to get more information. Asking questions like, "Is your throat sore?" to elicit a "yes or no" answer is not as productive and often leads to less information. Try for a mix of different questions to get all the information you can.

◈ ◈ ◈ ◈ ◈

Oh, I know what you must be thinking. How can you ever ask all these questions? This is too much work. Just grab the antihistamine, take the aspirin, and forget homeopathy!

I know this looks daunting, but professional homeopaths just let the person talk; they will tell you what is important. If you ask how he feels, he will do most of the work for you. Once your family gets a sense of what you are looking for, they will learn to report what they need to in order to get well.

In time, you will find your own style to elicit the information you need to know to treat colds and flu homeopathically.

In the next chapter, we will see how these questions work when you try to find a remedy for a cold. Trust me—it's really not as hard as it looks.

That's Why They Call It "Practicing":
Three Sample Cases

OK, by now, you're probably wondering what it's like to actually take a case. How much information are you supposed to get, how much will the person be likely to tell you? The answer is, considering the long list of what to watch out for, not much. The good news is, not much is enough.

Let's walk through three sample cases that might happen at your house. For example. . .

Case One:

After calling your teenager several times to come down and eat breakfast before he goes to school, you go to his room to find he is still in bed. This is not at all unusual--you have to drag him out of bed once a week or so. You shake him by the shoulder several times, but to no avail.

You: Get up!

Son: Uuugh.

You: What's wrong? Are you sick?

Son: I feel terrible.

(He sits up, and his face is flushed)

You: What's wrong?

Son: I don't feel good. I don't wanna go to school.

You: You'll have to do better than that.

(Despite your words, you can see his face is a little   red.)

Son: No, really, my throat is sore. I had bad dreams all night.

You: Too many horror movies.

Son: Bugs and spiders. My throat hurts every time I swallow.

You: Do you have a runny nose?

Son: No. But my head really hurts.

You: Where?

Son: My temples and the back of my head.

You: You were fine when you went to bed last
night.
Son: I know. I felt great. I almost didn't want to go
to bed, I was so wide-awake. Then I woke up
around two o'clock feeling terrible.
You: Are you achy, too?
Son: No, not really, just my head and throat.
You: Do you want to eat anything?
Son: What I want to do is drink. I'm really thirsty.
You: You want some orange juice?
Son: What I really want is lemonade. Do we have any? I
want to just drink and go to sleep.

◆ ◆ ◆ ◆ ◆

The next step is to take out the chart in the back of this
book, which I hope you have photocopied, and look up some
symptoms. Even though the exchange between you and your son
was short, you have gotten a lot of information. You have
discovered that:

1. The illness came on suddenly.
2. His face is a little red.
3. His throat is very sore.
4. His head hurts on the temples and in back.
5. He is not hungry.
6. He is thirsty.
7. He's thirsty for lemonade.
8. For an oncoming cold, he is dry. No nasal discharge, no
postnasal drip, etc.
9. Body aches are minimal.
10. He's had some nightmares, his sleep was disturbed.
11. He wants to sleep.

You might be able to look up "bugs" or "spiders" but at
least you can look up "nightmares." Take out a copy of the chart,
and list the symptoms on the top so you know what you're looking
up. Then look them up in the following way, remembering to add
an additional "check" for a keynote symptom marked with an

asterisk. I usually just list my extras in the far right columns. The repertory to look up symptoms is found at the end of this book.

> Onset: Sudden
> Face: Color: Red
> Throat: Painful: Very Painful (he mentioned it several times)
> Headache: Location: Temples
> Headache: Location: Back
> Appetite: No Appetite
> Food: Thirst
> Food: Thirst: Lemonade
> Sleep: Nightmares

Look up the symptoms you find. Your chart should look something like this when you have it finished:

	Sudden Onset	Face and Cheeks Red	Throat Painful	Headaches: Temple	Headaches: Back	No Appetite	Thirsty	Thirsty For Lemonade	Nightmares	Wants To Sleep				Extras
Aconitum	√	√								√				√
Allium Cepa							√							
Anas Barbar.														
Arsenicum						√								
Belladonna	√	√	√	√	√		√	√	√				√	√
Bryonia				√		√								
Calcarea Carb									√					
Eupatorium														
Euphrasia		√												
Ferrum Phos		√												
Gelsemium					√									
Hepar Sulph														
Influenzinum														
Kali Bichrom.							√							
Lycopodium		√					√							
Mercury									√					
Natrum Mur							√							
Nux Vomica					√	√	√			√				
Phosphorus									√	√				
Pulsatilla				√										
Rhus Tox						√	√							√
Sulphur														

Let's say under "sleep" you were not sure which category applied, so instead of being more specific you listed all that were better from sleep. That's OK!

Now, total up the symptoms. Did you come up with Belladonna? That's what I would pick. Remember that Belladonna is dry, red, and sudden.

Congratulations! You've done your first case. Now for another one.

◈   ◈   ◈   ◈   ◈

Your husband comes home from work early. He slams the car door when he gets out of the car, comes into the house, yells at the kids to be quiet, asks if there is any coffee as he goes up to change clothes. Sometimes he will come home cranky, but this has a sharp edge to it, even for him.

When he comes down to drink the coffee, you can see that he is a little congested.

You: Are you OK?

Him: (edgy) I'm fine.

You: You sound a little clogged up, is all.

Him: Yeah, my nose is stopped up.

You: What's coming out?

Him: Nothing. I just can't breathe. Kind of off and on, though.

You: How's your throat?

Him: Kind of sore.

You: Is it more sore on one side that the other? What about swallowing?

Him: It's about equal. But it hurts worse when I swallow.

You: Any headache?

Him: Yeah, on the right side.

You: Any earache?

Him: No. But the weird thing was that I had the worse indigestion and heartburn after lunch. We all went to Mario's (Mario's is the pasta place near the office). Usually it never bothers me, but this time, I really felt it.

You: When did it hit you?

Him: Around three o'clock. Boy, I'm beginning to feel bad. I'm too busy to get sick.
You: Is there anything else bothering you?
Him: No.
You: How many cups of coffee is this?
Him: (laughing) About twelve!

OK, in this short a time, you managed to find out the following symptoms:

1. He's a little irritable, maybe at noise.
2. His nose is stuffy and blocked.
3. His nose is blocked off and on.
4. His throat is sore, worse swallowing (you could have asked what kind of pain, but that's enough).
5. He has a right-sided headache.
6. He had indigestion and heartburn after eating.
7. He wanted spicy food at lunch.
8. He drank a lot of coffee.
9. He's feeling overworked.

Take out a remedy sheet, list the symptoms, and look them up. This is how you would look them up:

Mind: Irritable
Mind: Hypersensitive To Noise
Nose: Blocked
Nose: Blocked Off And On
Throat: Pain Worse Swallowing
Headache: Location: Right Side
Stomach: Upset: After A Meal
Food: Desires: Spicy
Heartburn: After A Meal
Food: Overindulgence: Coffee
Cause: Exhaustion/Overwork

This is what your chart would look like, after you marked it up, remembering to add an extra "check" for starred symptoms:

	Irritable	Sensitive To Noise	Nose Blocked	Nose Blocked: Off and On	Throat Worse Swallowing	Headache Right Side	Stomach Upset After Meal	Desires Spicy Food	Heartburn After Meal	Overindulgence Coffee	Exhaustion	Overwork			Extras
Aconitum															
Allium Cepa															
Anas Barbar.															
Arsenicum	√														
Belladonna					√										
Bryonia	√		√												√
Calcarea Carb							√			√					
Eupatorium															
Euphrasia															
Ferrum Phos	√				√							√			
Gelsemium	√														
Hepar Sulph	√							√							
Influenzinum															
Kali Bichrom.			√						√						
Lycopodium															
Mercury				√											
Natrum Mur															
Nux Vomica	√	√						√		√	√	√	√	√	√
Phosphorus				√				√							
Pulsatilla			√	√											
Rhus Tox						√						√			
Sulphur												√			

Notice that it's OK to mark more than one column in a category, such as the remedy for all the heartburn conditions, since you can't tell which would be best. Also, if you remember something about a remedy—such as Pulsatilla symptoms being changeable, it's OK to mark that too.

After you added it up, you came up with Nux Vomica, right? That would be my choice. You know he's overworked and craving stimulants. Often, that's all it takes.

◆ ◆ ◆ ◆ ◆

OK, ready for round three? Here goes:

Your four—year—old is normally a sweet little girl, able to play alone for long periods of time. But, you notice that for the last couple of days she's gotten really clingy, needs to be with you all the time, and cries when you try to leave her with the sitter. She's had a slight runny nose, and until today you didn't feel it was anything significant. Today, though, the discharge has gotten worse and now turned yellow. She's running a fever (99°). She has been coughing, sometimes dry, sometimes wet, even though there doesn't seem to be fluid in her lungs. She puts her hand to her ear occasionally. You decide it's time to get your kit of remedies out and see what you can do.

You: Do your ears hurt, honey?

She: No. They feel funny.

You: How?

She: I don't know.

You: Do you want something to eat?

She: Can I have peanut butter? I love peanut butter!

You: OK.

(You go to pick up her cup and see that she has left half of her orange juice, which she usually drinks by the quart, if not by the gallon.)

You: Are you thirsty? You want some more juice?

She: No.

You: How does your head feel? Does anything hurt?

She: My tummy, sometimes.

You: Is there anything else that's bothering you?

She: Nope.

❖ ❖ ❖ ❖ ❖

You might think that you couldn't get many symptoms out of a young child, but you've got some symptoms to work with. You can see that she's clingy and changeable; she's got a yellow nasal discharge, her cough is alternately dry and wet, she's not thirsty, she wants to eat peanut butter (that's about the eighth time she asked for it in three days). She can't say what the stomach pain is like.

Here's how you would look the symptoms up:

Mind: Company Ameliorates
Mind: Traits: Clingy
Nose: Discharge: Color of Discharge: Yellow
Cough: Dry
Cough: Wet
Food: Thirstless
Food: Desires: Peanut butter

The stomach pain you will leave off for now, since her symptoms are vague.

When you do the chart, it would look something like this:

	Wants Company	Clingy	Yellow Nasal Discharge	Dry Cough	Wet Cough	Not Thirsty	Desires Peanut Butter	Cough First Dry, Then Wet						Extras
Aconitum	√														
Allium Cepa															
Anas Barbar.															
Arsenicum															
Belladonna				√	√	√									
Bryonia															
Calcarea Carb			√												
Eupatorium															
Euphrasia					√										
Ferrum Phos															
Gelsemium						√									
Hepar Sulph			√												
Influenzinum															
Kali Bichrom.			√												√
Lycopodium						√									
Mercury															
Natrum Mur															
Nux Vomica						√									
Phosphorus	√							√							√
Pulsatilla	√	√				√	√								√
Rhus Tox															
Sulphur			√		√										

Did you come up with Pulsatilla? I would have. She wants company, the nasal discharge is yellow, the cough is changing all the time, and she's got a desire for creamy foods. When you add the ear symptom into the mix, Pulsatilla would be a safe bet. You did it again!

See how far you have come? Sure, it would be better if your family were more verbal and you really could get more questions answered. A perfect case would include what makes a sore throat better or worse, what a pain *really* feels like, when the fever peaks, and other specific symptoms. These all would be valuable clues to the right remedy. But, there will be times when you can't get that information, either because the person is not verbal enough, has not learned to articulate how they feel, or—let's face it—you forget. Just do the best you can, which will be good enough.

Now, let's see how the remedies work and how to take them once you have figured which one fits the case.

How Remedies Work

Homeopaths believe that illness has an unseen, dynamic cause and hence, an unseen, dynamic cure. However, with the advance of physics in the 20th century, it seems that we are now closer to understanding how the remedies work than we were a hundred years ago.

Einstein, in his equation $E=MC^2$, made us all aware that matter and energy are the same. Matter may be turned into energy or vice versa. This equation underscored a relationship between the two that has helped us conceptualize how remedies work. It shows us how energy built up in the dilution and succussion process changes the substance so that it is more suited to affecting the vital force.

There has also been some speculation, fully covered in George Vithoulkas's book *The Science of Homeopathy,* that remedies work because their atomic vibration is close to the vibration of the sick person.[3] The disease itself makes the person susceptible to the vibrations of the right remedy, and the closer a "fit" the remedy vibration is, the more the patient will react to it. Therefore, it's possible to help a cold even though the remedy is not an exact fit. Remedies taken at the wrong time have no effect on the patient because the resonance between the person and that remedy at that time is not aclose match.

Because the remedies are diluted and sucussed, they seem to work on an atomic level. Researchers have found that there is a magnetic component to the brain, called "Magnetite. We don't know *why* it is there, we only know it *is* there. There has been some thought that remedies may work on this magnetic component.

---

3 George Vithoulkas, *The Science Of Homeopathy,* (New York: Grove Weidenfeld, 1981), p. 75ff.

These theories may be interesting, but what we absolutely know about homeopathic remedies is they are truly "holistic" because they treat the body, mind, and spirit at the same time with the same dose. They are efficacious for chronic illness as well as the acute cold or flu, and it is the purpose of this book to help you find the best "fit" of the remedies included.

In order to treat colds and flu effectively, I have to tell you how remedies work. It will help you determine your next step in treating colds or flu.

❖ ❖ ❖ ❖ ❖

Remedies work in two major ways: aggravation and amelioration. This is a fancy way of saying the person either gets worse (temporarily) or he gets better.

Remember Herring's law of cure? When a person is cured, the first part of the body to get better is the vital force—which we can see as the energy level—or mental symptoms. Also, the last symptom he got will be the first symptom to be relieved, or he gets better first in a more important part of his body, then a less important, than a lesser important, and so on, until he is cured.

Let's say you have a child with a cold. The first symptom was a sore throat followed by sneezing. He carried on for a few days saying that nothing was wrong, but now he has started running a fever. Finally he became so lethargic he could scarcely get out of bed. He now has got a copious yellow discharge from his nose.

You give him a remedy—let's say it's Pulsatilla—and although he still has got a terrible runny nose, and still having bouts of sore throat when he talks a lot, he is up and out of bed and planning to go to school. His energy level is a little higher, which is how you know the remedy is working. It should eventually clear up the other symptoms, if the symptoms remain the same until they are relieved. Remember, what you are looking for is change which usually starts with mental symptoms or with the patient's energy level.

It is very common for people with a cold to complain that they aren't getting any better because there has been no decrease in the amount of nasal discharge, coughing, etc. But what's important is to watch them to see if their level of activity, their energy, their vital force has gotten better or stayed the same.

Remember, too, that we are talking about voluntary activity. An adult who forces himself out of bed to go to work may not have a real increase in the vital force, but may only be doing it out of duty and strength of will. But if you look at voluntary activity, what you would see might be something like this:

Monday: Ate part of two meals, read for one hour, dozed or slept the rest of the day.

Tuesday: Ate two meals, read for two hours, watched a movie on TV, talked with friend on phone for 15 minutes.

Wednesday: Ate three meals, went to market for soup, talked with friend on the phone for an hour, changed sheets on bed, washed hair.

You can see that the general progression is on an upward trend. More and more voluntary activities are being done and the patient is sleeping less. This is an amelioration of the cold, and he is getting better.

◈ ◈ ◈ ◈ ◈

The second way a remedy can work is by aggravation. Aggravation is what happens when the remedy given is too high for the person's body chemistry. Aggravations may happen as a result of prescribing, but they also occur because oftentimes a person's disease would resonate best to a remedy in a potency between two that are made. There is no chemical law that your cold would necessarily respond best to a potency you have been given. For example, what a person might really need is a 35C remedy instead of a 30 C. Although it is possible to make a 35C it is not a potency that is available. The person's illness may fit perfectly a potency that is not made.

What may happen when a potency is given that is too high is an aggravation. The person's symptoms may get a little worse temporarily, nasal secretions may increase. Another thing that may happen is that the person may develop another symptom that is associated with that remedy but that he did not have before—for example, with Arsenicum, he may become uncharacteristically chilly right after taking the remedy.

Because you will be using mostly 30C remedies for a cold, a low potency, aggravations are rare. Although it is sometimes hard for even professional homeopaths to distinguish an aggravation from the normal progression of a disease, there are several ways to tell:

1. The person got worse immediately after taking the remedy.

2. The symptoms he developed are consistent with the remedy he took.

3. Even though some symptoms are worse, his energy level is higher.

4. Even though his symptoms are worse, he is calmer about his illness than he was before.

If it is an aggravation, it will be followed by a quick rebound and the person is better than he was before he took the remedy. Once again, your cold is on the way to getting better.

Another pattern emerges if the remedy was given in too low a dose. When this happens the repeated doses partially make up for the dose being too low. The cold will get better for a short while, but the improvement does not hold and he begins to slip back. In that case, it would be better to put the remedy in water as discussed in the chapter "Time To Take Your Medicine." Putting the remedy in water makes it a little stronger and the dose changes slightly every time you stir it. Often, that's all it takes to finish off your cold.

Time To Take Your Medicine

After you have figured out what remedy the person needs, you can order the remedy through one of the pharmacies listed in the back of this book or, if you have chosen a 30C potency or less, you can probably find it in the nearest good-sized health food store.

If you do order the remedy through mail order, make sure you order it from a reputable long-established homeopathic pharmacy. The best size to order is a 2 dram bottle, which will give you enough to have at home for future use. Your remedies will come to you in the form of small granules. We usually order what is called a "number 10 pellet" which is the smallest size granule. We find that a bottle lasts longer, taking only 12-15 granules at a time. If the pharmacy doesn't have that small a size, just order the smallest size pellet they stock. If you have ordered bigger granules, don't despair—just take two per dose, and that should be enough.

If you buy the remedies in a health food store, you may buy something that is a small tablet, similar to a baby aspirin. Those will work just fine, although I think, over the long term, they will crumble if they are carried around in your purse or in your luggage too long.

There are books to tell you what remedies follow the others well in treatment for chronic or deep-seated illness. (Homeopaths call these deep-seated cases that involve deeper organs "constitutional cases.") However, for the treatment of colds and flu, I just need to say one thing about the order of remedies. Lycopodium Clavatum does not follow Sulphur well. If you do take Lycopodium Clavatum after Sulphur, it will not make you acutely ill, but you will feel out of sorts. If you take Sulphur for a cold and then see that Lycopodium Clavatum would have been a better choice, take another remedy before you take the Lycopodium Clavatum. Calcarea works particularly well with both Sulphur and Lycopodium. Always take a Calcarea Carbonica dose of the same strength as the previous Sulphur dose. This should work fine.

The other remedy to be careful with is Sulphur. If someone has advanced tuberculosis, he should not take high dose Sulphur.

After you purchase the remedy and are ready to give it (or take it, if it's for yourself) there are several simple rules and procedures you need to follow in order to make taking the remedies most effective:

1. Never touch the remedies with your hands. Shake out one or two granules, in the case of the larger ones, or ten to fifteen tiny ones, into the cap of the bottle, hold your breath, and toss them in your mouth. Be careful not to touch the inside of the cap, touch the cap to your mouth, or sneeze, cough, or breathe into the cap. Put the cap back on tightly.

Some remedies have a twist cap vial that disperses several into the cap. That is perfectly OK; just follow these same rules so you won't contaminate the contents.

2. Wait twenty to thirty minutes before and after taking the remedies to eat or drink anything. Water is safe, but all other beverages must wait. Also, wait twenty to thirty minutes before and after brushing your teeth, chewing gum, or having anything in your mouth, except water.

3. The remedies will work better if you do not drink coffee or smoke. If you simply can not give up these things, try to cut back as much as possible, and try not to have the coffee or cigarette until just before your next dose, in order to give the remedy maximum time to work. Please note that it is not the caffeine that is the problem; it is the coffee bean itself. Colas and tea are fine to drink in moderation, the exception being Earl Grey tea, which contains another possible remedy antidote.

4. Keep the remedies away from all electrical appliances; don't put them on top of or next to phones, computers, televisions, electronic organizers, on top of the dishwasher or washer and dryer. For more tips, see the chapter, "How To Take Care Of Your Remedies."

5. Don't spray cleaning solutions near the remedies, or keep them near any strong smelling substance. Most people keep them in a dresser drawer, if they do not have scented paper or potpourri in them. Kitchen cabinets work well if they are not lined with pesticide—treated shelf paper.

It's important to keep yourself or your patient away from strong smells as well. *Do not* use camphor, menthol, or eucalyptus preparations while giving someone else a remedy or taking one yourself. Remember that they do not have to be on you to antidote you; if your spouse drenches himself or herself in this stuff before bedtime, it will antidote you as well.

If you happen to paint or wallpaper your house, double or triple bag the remedies in airtight food storage bags and keep them at the other end of the house, as far away from the work area as you can get them.

6. If you take more than one dose of the same potency remedy, it may work better if you mix it in water. To do this, put the remedy into one-quarter to one-half a cup of bottled water. Distilled water is best; do not use tap water. Stir it, take a teaspoon of the water, and cover the cup so that it can remain undisturbed. *Do not* put the teaspoon that was in your mouth back in the water. Use a fresh teaspoon each time.

This solution will only last for 24 hours. At the end of that time, throw it away. If you still need to take the remedy, make a fresh batch.

7. The remedies will keep working after you take the last dose, so there is usually no need to keep taking a remedy until you are completely well. Stop taking the remedy when you are fifty to sixty percent better. If you don't remain better, go back to the remedy or go up one potency level—usually a 200C—and see if that brings more lasting relief.

8. Occasionally, if someone takes a remedy too frequently or the dose was too strong, he may experience an "aggravation" a temporary worsening of the original symptoms or a new symptom belonging to that same remedy. For example, let's say you are giving your son, age six, Pulsatilla for a cold. You notice that after several doses he becomes increasingly more clingy and demanding of your attention. If you look up Pulsatilla you will see that clinging and craving attention are mental symptoms of Pulsatilla and he is having a slight aggravation.

The correct thing to do is stop taking the remedy for a day or two. If the aggravation is bothersome enough, you may want to give a dose of Nux Vomica, which antidotes many remedies, or a cup of coffee. Be aware though, that if you do antidote the remedy by one of these means, you will also stop the beneficial aspects of the remedy. It would be best, then, to wait, and do nothing rather than undo the good it has done.

The good news is that these aggravations are usually minor and are always temporary. The even better news is that, since people do not aggravate from the wrong remedy, an aggravation ensures that the remedy was correct and the person will get better.

When in doubt, you can always contact the nearest homeopathic practitioner. If you don't know anyone, the National Center For Homeopathy should be able to put you in touch with someone in your area.

❖ ❖ ❖ ❖ ❖

That's all you need to know about taking the remedies. I hope you meet with great success. But if you don't. . .

What Am I Doing Wrong?

When Homeopathy Doesn't Work

Every since Hahnemann kept a bottle of Spirits of Ammonia to give to patients when he wanted to blunt or slow down the action of the remedies, there has been an ongoing discussion about what substances keep the remedies from working. There are as many views of this as there are homeopaths, and it is not at all unusual for a patient who has used homeopathy for many years to have various practitioners disagree about what he should and shouldn't do. Just be aware as you read this chapter that what I am reporting is as general a view as I can give.

Even professional homeopaths don't have a one-hundred-percent success rate. The good news is that even when your remedies don't work for a cold and flu, they are at least saving you from taking other things that might interfere with the cold and create other problems. Each day without a nasal decongestant is another day you are not risking dependence on them. Each day without unnecessary antibiotics is insurance against the day when your life may depend on taking them and, because of not overusing them, you are not drug resistant. Each trip to the doctor's office avoided means that you are not exposed to microbes which you would seldom encounter in your normal day.

But, even with these benefits, taking a remedy and seeing no improvement is exasperating. There are several reasons why homeopathy may not work for your specific case of cold or flu. Here's what those reasons are:

The most common problem is that you are eating, drinking or brushing your teeth too close to the time you are taking the remedies. Remember to follow, or have your family follow, the twenty to thirty minute rule: wait twenty to thirty minutes after you eat or drink, take the remedy, and then wait twenty to thirty minutes before you eat or drink. Breaking this rule will make it harder for the remedies to work.

Remember not to rush in too soon with another remedy before deciding that the previous one does not work. Please give each remedy enough time to work, by taking at least several doses, before you reevaluate if you should continue with your original choice.

Also, check to see if you are around any of the substances that interfere with remedies. To repeat what was covered in Chapter five, there are three major offenders: camphor, menthol, and eucalyptus. These substances are found in a lot of common preparations, among them body rubs like BenGay or Tiger Balm. Cold preparations like Vick's Vap-O-Rub are filled with them, as are some hair shampoos, most nail polishes, shaving creams, and of course, cigarettes.

Not only do you have to keep them off *yourself*, you have to keep them away from the remedies themselves. By "keep away" I mean that the remedies should be at the *other end of the house* from these substances. For most people, this means that the medicine chest is the *worst* place for homeopathic remedies and should be avoided. For this reason, a lot of people keep their remedies in a clothes closet, which is fine as long as there is no camphor in the closet, or in a kitchen cabinet or dresser drawer. Remember, too, that these substances need not be on *you* to antidote you. If your spouse drenches him/herself in mentholatum before bed, you will want to find a better solution for them at the health food store before you treat yourself for a cold or flu homeopathically.

There are several other chemicals that may antidote remedies, for example, chlorine and mint, especially peppermint. Occasionally we have noticed that some people antidote the action of the remedies when they swim in heavily chlorinated pools in the summer, or, when they brush their teeth with strong toothpaste. Of course, most people can swim in a chlorinated pool with no problem, although we suggest that they not swim on or near the day the pool is treated if it is treated on a weekly or monthly basis. And, although some homeopaths believe that peppermint antidotes remedies, we have found, except for very strong peppermint candies, mint generally is not a sizable problem for most people. But if you are avoiding camphor, menthol, and eucalyptus, and your remedy is still not working, then consider avoiding these two substances as well.

One of the biggest impediments to homeopathic treatment is smoking. While it's true that a lot of homeopaths refuse to treat patients who smoke because chances of success are diminished, every homeopath has treated a smoker and achieved results. If you have only an occasional cigarette and can give up the habit during the time you have the cold, so much the better. And, if you can stop smoking altogether, not only will you add years to your life but make another alternative for help open to you.

There are other habits that will interfere with homeopathic remedies. One of the most common is drinking coffee, which will antidote most remedies. Please remember that it is not the caffeine in the coffee that will antidote you, it's something in the coffee bean itself. Therefore, decaffeinated coffee is not acceptable either. Even coffee flavoring, such as in candy or ice cream, may antidote a remedy. While coffee may not antidote *your* particular remedy, it's a good habit not to drink coffee while you are treating yourself. However, homeopaths do disagree on this issue, some being more liberal and allowing coffee, some allowing coffee depending on the type of remedy. My motto has always been "better safe than sorry." If your remedy is not working, cut out the coffee.

Another controversial idea is whether or not sleeping under an electric blanket will antidote remedies. Many homeopaths believe that the electric energy field of an electric blanket will interfere with remedy action; others are concerned that most people will set the temperature setting too high and wake up frying. Certainly, it must be healthier simply to put another blanket on the bed. If you really have a problem keeping your body temperature stable when sleeping, please see your physician or a professional homeopath.

Another item of controversy is drugs. Some practitioners prefer not to treat clients who take prescription drugs daily. However, many practitioners find that usually a drug's actions are too crude to affect homeopathic treatment. In general, people do better taking the remedies and their prescription drugs than relying on prescription drugs alone. In treatment of colds and flu, we usually tell people it's all right to take aspirin or Tylenol. In my experience, however, antihistamines usually do more harm than good, creating an unhealthy dependency.

So in sum, if your remedy is not working, look for hidden sources of camphor, menthol, eucalyptus, coffee, chlorine, mint, or electrical currents, either in or on you, someone near you, or near your remedies.

Another frequently asked question is whether other methods of treatment can be used concurrently with homeopathy. For example, Victor McCabe says that mixing acupuncture and homeopathy does not work well. He prefers clients try homeopathy for a while and then switch to acupuncture, then go back to homeopathy. However, we have found in our practice that many people benefit from using acupuncture and homeopathy concurrently.

Bach flower remedy potencies can be used with high dose remedies, remedies higher than you would use for colds and flu. If you use Bach remedies, it is better to suspend them while using other remedies to treat your cold or flu.

Homeopathic remedies should not be used with aromatherapy, because of the heavy use of menthol and camphor. Also questionable is to use herbal remedies with homeopathic ones. Many homeopaths will not treat people who insist on taking herbal preparations concurrently, because the herbal substances are medicinal in themselves. Other homeopaths feel that the herbs are in too crude a dose to interfere with the remedies. We find, in general, that herbal preparations may provide relief, but they do not achieve permanent improvements in health like homeopathic ones do.

Check the chapter "How To Take Care Of Your Remedies" to see if your remedy is at fault. Radiation from an airport security metal detector will neutralize remedies. Make sure, when you travel, that the remedies are not x-rayed, or they will be rendered worthless.

In a more logical world, these rules would apply to all patients equally. Some rules, like the one about camphor, seem to be true all the time. Other rules, like the coffee rule, can sometimes be bent. Can some people drink coffee and still have the remedy work? Are some people especially sensitive to peppermint? Is it possible to use Goldenseal along with homeopathic Pulsatilla? Of course. These rules depend on the remedy, the person, and the illness involved. But I think it is better to be careful and follow the rules, than to break them and then have to wonder if the remedy is the correct, or, indeed, if homeopathy works for you at all.

There are other more subtle reasons that the remedies might not work. The first factor is not that common for acute cases like colds or flu, but it is worth mentioning nevertheless. In cases where the illness is due to some environmental stress or job condition that cannot be changed, homeopathy may prove ineffective. For example, the person who has frequent colds because his desk is right under the air conditioning vent at work may not cut back on his cold frequency until the desk is moved.

Another impediment to healing is often the patient's lifestyle. Many people who have a cold think that they can go about their lives in the usual way or even an accelerated manner. Late hours, alcohol consumption, overwork, poor diet, not drinking enough fluids—lifestyle choices like these can influence how long a cold lasts and make it almost impossible for a remedy to work. Remember to give your body a reasonable chance to heal itself.

And one last mention of a healing impediment: if one is receiving secondary gains from frequent colds, such as the attention a child gets from a too-busy parent, then the child may still get colds despite treatment. The secondary gain has to be dealt with before healing can occur.

Although homeopathy is not mind over matter, and it works whether the person believes in it or not, it is also true that people who don't want to believe in homeopathy will deny their progress and often sabotage and impede their own treatment. For this reason it is hard to treat someone who categorically does not believe in homeopathy or is not open to alternative methods of treatment.

All these subtle conditions may effect your success.

Luckily, these conditions are relatively rare. After a discussion of two common over-the-counter products, the next section, a Homeopathic *Materia Medica*, lists the symptoms associated with the most common cold and flu remedies. I hope you find it interesting.

Too Busy A Case To Try?
Buy These Remedies On The Fly!

Sometimes, life crowds in on us and there is just no way we can spare the time to do a case properly and find the exact remedy. In my personal experience, there are two products sold in many health food or drug stores that will mitigate your cold or flu. So here is a brief description of them, with supporting evidence of their efficacy, for you to try when you are just too busy to utilize this book fully.

❖ ❖ ❖ ❖ ❖

The most popular flu remedy in France and growing in popularity in the United States is a remedy with an almost unpronounceable name: Oscillococcinum (O-sill-o-cox-see-num). Sold in packages of three or six tubes, it's often the first remedy a homeopathy newcomer tries when faced with colds or flu.

There have been several studies that have shown the efficacy of Oscillococcinum. One was published in the British Journal of Clinical Pharmacology in 1989 and conducted by J. P. Ferley, D. Zmirou, D. D'adhemar and F. Balducci.[4] It was composed of 237 patients who received Oscillococcinum and 241 who were given a placebo composed of the lactose and sucrose in the remedy but no Anas Barbarae, the active ingredient. The patients recorded their rectal temperatures twice a day, and reported the presence or absence of five cardinal symptoms: headache, stiffness, lumbar and articular (joint) pain, and shivers.

---

[4]J.P. Ferley, D. Zmirou, D. d'Adémar, and F. Balducci, "A Controlled Evaluation Of a Homeopathic Preparation In the Treatment of Influenza-like Syndromes," *British Journal Of Clinical Pharmacology*, (1989; 27): pp. 329-335.

Many also had a cough, coryza (runny nose) and fatigue. Patients had to be 12 years or older, with rectal temperatures of 38°C (100.4°F) or higher, and at least two of the above symptoms. Patients who had flu shots or a history of depression were excluded. Patients were asked not to take anything for fever, or if they did, record what they took.

Recovery was judged with a temperature less than 37.5°C (99.5°F) and cessation of the five cardinal symptoms above. Of those who took the placebo, only 10.3% were relieved of symptoms versus 17.1 of those who received Oscillococcinum.

◆ ◆ ◆ ◆ ◆

Ferley's study was replicated by Rosemarie Papp, Gert Schuback, Elmar Beck, George Berkard, Jorgen Bengel, Siegfried Lehrl, and Philippe Belon in the British Homeopathic Journal.5

Their criterion for cure was that rectal temperature had to be 38°C (100.4°F) or less. Their patients, between the ages of 12 and 60, did not have prior flu shots, nor did they take other medication within the 48 hours of trial.

Finally, there were 167 patients in both valid groups who had taken either the Oscillococcinum or the placebo.

Forty-eight hours after treatment, they accessed the patients' compliance and their fitness for work. At the end of the study, 19.2% of the verum (remedy) group had no symptoms and 43.7% had clearly improved. In the placebo group, only 15% had no symptoms and only 33% had clear improvement. In addition, although 5.4% of the placebo group had gotten worse by the end of 48 hours, none of the Oscillococcinum group deteriorated. The study concluded that it "economically made sense" to take the Oscillococcinum, as those who took the remedy missed less work.

Another study published in 1984 in the French magazine *Tonus* by Professor Casanova and Drs. Basquin, Mangennay, Pacotte and Questel in 1984 describe another double bind study

---

5Rosemarie Papp. Gert Schuback, Elmar Beck, Georg Burkard, Jurgen Bengel, Siegfried Lehrl and Philippe Belon, "Oscillococcinum In Patients With Influenza-like Syndromes: A Placebo-Controlled Double-Blind Evaluation, *British Homoeopathic Journal*. (April 1998, vol. 87), pp. 69-76.

with volunteers who took Oscillococcinum within 48 hours of onset. Again, patients on antibiotics or who had flu shots were excluded. They took four doses a day for shivering, aches and pains, rhinorrhea (runny nose) and coughing and fever. It seemed to work best for runny noise and bronchial congestion when it was taken early.

All of these studies seem to reinforce the efficacy of Oscillococcinum, or Anas Barbarae, as I have listed it in this book under its remedy name. However you pronounce it, don't forget it at cold and flu time for a fast pick for indicated symptoms.

◈ ◈ ◈ ◈ ◈

Another useful remedy is Zicam, a product of Matrixx Initiatives, the manufacturer of almost a dozen cold and allergy products. The flagship remedy, Zicam cold remedy nasal gel, is a homeopathic preparation of Zinc marketed in an application bottle or in swabs sized for children and adults.

As with Oscillococcinum, studies have been published showing the efficacy of Zicam. The first study of zinc nasal gel seems to be an unpublished study by C. B. Hensley, Ph.D. and Davidson, Ph.D. in 1999.[6]

Subsequently, three researchers, Michael Hirt, MD, Sion Nobel, MD, and Ernesto Barron, BS, performed a double bind, placebo-controlled trial of Zicam to see if they could repeat the results of the earlier study.

They began with 213 patients. All patients had to have a recent onset of cold symptoms, within the last 24 hours. The investigators required participants to have at least three of the following symptoms: cough, headache, hoarseness, muscle ache, nasal drainage, nasal congestion, scratchy throat, sore throat, or sneezing. Conditions that would exclude a patient from participating were pregnancy, any condition that would compromise his or her auto immune system, onset of symptoms

---

[6]Michael Hirt, MD, Sion Nobel, MD, Ernesto Barron, BS, "Zinc Nasal Gel For the Treatment Of Common Cold Symptoms: A Double-blind, Placebo-controlled Trial", *ENT: Ear Nose and Throat Journal*, (October, 2000, vol. 79, Number 10).

longer than 24 hours previously, and the use of certain medications. One hundred and eight patients received the Zicam, and one hundred and five received placebo, a gel exactly like Zicam but with no zinc.

The results were dramatic: duration of the cold for the Zicam Patients was only 2.3 days, versus nine days for those taking the identical but inert placebo. It was clear that Zicam helped the cold.

Also encouraging was the fact that, although patients in both the placebo and zinc groups reported a slight burning or tingling of the nose, none reported any common side effects of other cold medications, such as nausea, bad taste reactions, odor, dizziness, and drowsiness.

These results were similar to those of a later study by S. B. Mossad, From the Cleveland Clinic Foundation.[7]

They studied 80 patients, half of which received Zinc nasal gel and the other half receiving a placebo. Unlike the previous study, they accepted patients who had the cold longer than twenty-four but up to forty-eight hours. Therefore, there would be at least one day's difference in the data. This study also differed in that symptoms were classified as either major or minor. Major symptoms were nasal drainage and sore throat, minor symptoms were: nasal congestion, sneezing, scratchy throat, hoarseness, cough, headache, muscle aches, and a fever of more than 98.6°F. After excluding conditions that would invalidate the study, such as pregnancy, recurrent sinusitis, or bronchitis, they also excluded patients who were using other cold remedies or who had ever used Zicam.

Patients and interviewers had no way of knowing if they were being given Zicam or a placebo. As in the earlier study, they took the Zicam four times a day.

Mossad found the zinc gel patients had an average duration of the cold 4.3 days versus six days for the placebo group. Some of this time discrepancy could be explained because this study accepted patients who had been sicker longer, and the Zicam

---

[7]S. B. Mossad, "Effect Of Zincum Gluconicum Nasal Gel On the Duration and Symptom Severity Of the Common Cold In Otherwise Healthy Adults", *QJM: Monthly Journal Of the Association Of Physicians*, (vol. 96, number 1, 2003), pp.35-43.

directions state that it works best when taken early. He found that duration of hoarseness, sore throat, nasal drainage and nasal congestion were significantly shorter in the zinc group, however, the duration of sneezing and scratchy throats was not changed. He did remark that all symptoms were significantly milder for those taking the zinc gel.

These studies support my own experience with Zicam; it can be a powerful aid to dealing with a cold, and often is the difference between getting a full night's sleep or lying in bed, exhausted and sleepless, too stuffed up to breathe.

◈ ◈ ◈ ◈ ◈

And, as long as I am discussing helpful materials for newcomers to homeopathy, I have to mention Kent Homeopathic Associates. For those of you who are more comfortable with a computer than a book, they specialize in computer software on homeopathy. They offer MacRepertory, a complete repertory of all physical symptoms (not just one for colds and flu, which follows in this book), a complete materia medica of all remedies, and hundreds of ancient and modern books about homeopathy, all in colorful and easy-to-use programs for both Macintosh and PC systems. For those of you who want to continue learning homeopathy after you use this book, they will be happy to send you information about their programs. You will find them listed with other resources at the end of this book.

But, until you are ready to forage ahead, my advice is: when you are too busy to utilize this book, at least stop for five minutes to buy Oscillococcinum or Zicam, two remedies I have found useful for the treatment of colds and flu.

Part Three:

A COLD AND FLU

MATERIA MEDICA

Please note: categories with no symptoms
are marked with a "Ø"

Aconitum Napellus
(ack-con-eye-tum nay-pell-us)

The first remedy I want to talk about is Aconitum Napellus, or Aconite, and you will be successful in choosing Aconite if you keep two things in mind.

First, people who need Aconite for a cold are usually those who have caught a cold from exposure to a dry, cold wind or cold weather.

The practitioner must be careful not to take that statement too literally. For example, it is also common to develop an Aconite cold after some exertion outdoors, such as gardening. The person breaks into a sweat, perspires, and feels pretty good until the evening breeze springs up and he or she gets chilled. For this reason Aconite is associated with colds when the weather is especially hot and people are active outdoors. I myself have taken an Aconite cold when, at the end of summer, I accompanied a friend out to the apartment pool to watch her kids swim. We only sat by the pool and talked, but the breeze sprang up and, in combination with the cooler air from the pool, gave me a cold which Aconite cleared up quite quickly.

Secondly, in order for Aconite to be effective, you must take it at the first sign of a cold or flu. If you have any suspicion at all that the cold might be the result of exposure to wind, it's better to go ahead and give Aconite first, then follow it with another remedy if it fails to act. By *early*, I mean within the first 12-18 hours of symptoms. After that, the cold has changed to a different pattern and Aconite usually doesn't help.

Aconite, along with Coffea and Chamomilla, is considered a major homeopathic pain reliever. Aconite is also valuable for the effects of shock; it's a great remedy for car accidents or other trauma.

Another clear indicator of needing Aconite is fear, especially fear with restlessness. Children who need this remedy may become more fearful, especially at night. Patients are easily startled. They feel as though everything must be done in haste.

Hahnemann discovered Aconite in 1805. Both Aconite and Belladonna are poisonous in their natural states. Aconite's poison alkaloid is called "aconitine." Aconite is very similar to Belladonna—they both fit significant, if not violent, illnesses, which strike quickly.

Because of the suddenness of the Aconite cold and the imperative of acting quickly, it's a good choice to take along on a vacation; it's a lot easier to stop a cold before it really gets started than it is to treat a full blown cold.

Aconite has a brief action; therefore, if you think it is helping, you can repeat it more frequently than you might other remedies, taking it every three instead of every four hours for the first several doses.

❖ ❖ ❖ ❖ ❖

When considering Aconitum Napellus, think of the following:
  ✓ Exposure to dry cold wind
  ✓ Exposure to wind after perspiring
  ✓ Sudden onset
  ✓ Fearfulness
  ✓ Early stages of cold or flu
  ✓ Exposure to cold wind or temperature with illness the same day

❖ ❖ ❖ ❖ ❖

Other symptoms of Aconitum Napellus:

Cause: Fright or shock; chill; heat of sun; injury; surgery

Mind: Fearful; anxiety for no reason; fear of future or having hair cut; fear of crowds, flying, earthquakes; wants company; claustrophobia; feels as if he might die

Head: Head may be heavy, hot, pulsating; dizziness on rising or moving the head; headache feels like the head is being squeezed; burning hot head made worse by movement; pressure and headache is worse talking, when sitting up, and stooping

Face: Red face or alternately pale and then red

Eyes: Red, dry and hot, feels as if eyes have sand in them; may be adverse to light; eyelids swollen, hot, red; profuse tearing; specks in front of eyes; either light sensitive or wants lots of light

Ears: Ringing, buzzing, roaring in ears; tinnitus; ear pain after being out in severe cold; hypersensitive to noise; (music is unbearable); outer ear can be hot, red, swollen, or painful; better for warm applications

Nose: Either dry stuffiness with no sneezing with scanty watery discharge; or lots of discharge with dripping of clear hot water; sense of smell may be very acute; lots of sneezing; nose bleeds with bright red blood

Mouth and Tongue: Lip of tongue tingles; tongue coated white or yellow-white; dry mouth

Throat: Dark red, burning and stinging; tingling; tonsils swollen and dry; feeling of pain and constriction on swallowing

Larynx: Windpipe aches when breathing in; burning and pricking in the larynx; hoarseness

Neck and Back: Sensation as if back is bruised; stiff nape of neck, hip joints, and pelvis

Chest: Tightness in chest; stitching pain when breathing; breath hot; feels hard to breathe; short of breath

Cough: Short dry cough with tickling in throat; cough caused by cold wind; cough is worse when eating, drinking, or lying down; short dry cough with tickling in throat worse from tobacco smoke or emotional upset; whistling cough; constant dry cough; loud cough; wakes up with dry, loose, or croupy cough; spits nothing up, or sputum might be blood streaked

Extremities: Numbness and tingling in the arms and legs may be present; shooting pains in hip and knee; sweating, icy cold palms of hands; the hands may be hot with cold feet

Stomach: Ø

Food: Thirsty for large quantities of cold water; everything tastes bitter except water

Sleep: Restless at night; wakes with anxiety; lies on back with hand under head; can't sleep on side or sleeps sitting up; dreams and nightmares

Fever: Useful in beginning stage of fever; fever comes on suddenly and violently after chill; easily chilled when unwrapped; cold chills pass through him; alternating cold and hot; head burns but rest of body cold; the skin is hot and dry; fever peaks at 9:00 in the evening

Worse: Worse lying on right side; drinking cold water; interrupted sleep; exposure to tobacco smoke; at night; after midnight; in stuffy or warm room; in cold, dry wind

Better: In fresh or open air, after sleeping

Generals: Skin and senses oversensitive; restlessness; chilly; worse when listening to music; he demands that something must be done about his illness; profuse perspiration with anxiety; skin dry; heart palpitations

Allium Cepa
(al-lee-um see-pa)

If you have ever chopped onions, you have a pretty good idea of the use of Allium Cepa for a cold. This remedy is made from red onions, and you already know what they do: your eyes tear, your eyes get red, your nose runs. These symptoms all point to using Allium Cepa for a cold.

The major pointer for using Allium Cepa is to think of Allium Cepa and Euphrasia Officinalis as opposites. In Allium Cepa, the eyes tear and are red, but the tears are bland—they don't burn your face. It's the nasal discharge that burns; it often burns the edges of the nose, or under it. The other remedy, Euphrasia Officinalis, has the opposite symptom: eyes tear, but it's the tears that burn, while the nasal discharge is bland. It's easy to see why one of the first questions you are going to ask with any cold is: Is either the nasal discharge or tears from the eyes burning or reddening the skin?

People get Allium Cepa colds from cold, wet weather. They often get headaches in the forehead, resulting from the sinus congestion. They are often worse at the end of the day.

Allium Cepa might be a good pick if you are not sure if what you have is a cold or hay fever, as it is also a good treatment for hay fever, the other remedy being Arsenicum Album.

❖ ❖ ❖ ❖ ❖

Think of Allium Cepa if you see:
   ✓ Nasal discharge burning under the nose or sides of nose
   ✓ Any connection with hay fever or seasonal allergies
   ✓ Nasal congestion with headache in forehead
   ✓ Better outdoors, after cold rain

❖ ❖ ❖ ❖ ❖

Other symptoms of Allium Cepa include:

Cause: Exposure to damp, cold weather; spring colds; hay fever

Mind: Ø

Head: Headache, mostly in the forehead; pain in right temple

Face: Ø

Eyes: Itching and stinging eyes; profuse, bland tearing; red eyes; tendency to rub; eyes sensitive to light

Ears: Earache, shooting pain in the Eustachian tubes (especially in children); discharge of pus from ears

Nose: Sensitive to odor of peach skins and flowers; lots of watery discharge; nose burns; burning nasal discharge; constant and hearty sneezing; discharge may shift from side to side, one nostril drips at a time; discharge starts in left nostril and moves to the right; nasal discharge stops in open air and starts again in a warm room; pain wiping nose; tingling in nose

Mouth and Tongue: Top of lip sore

Throat: Red; hot; dry; tight; sensation of lump in throat

Larynx: Early stages of laryngitis or hoarseness; coughing hurts the larynx

Neck and Back: Pain at nape of neck; chills down back

Fever: Sweats easily and profusely

Chest: Cold may go to chest with lots of phlegm

Cough: Hacking cough when breathing in cold air; coughs from cold, damp, penetrating winds; croup, whooping cough, or bronchitis

Extremities: Ø

Stomach: Ø

Food: Thirsty; desire for raw onions; aversion to cucumbers

Sleep: Yawning, wakes at 2:00 in the morning; dreams of being near water, cliffs, storms, or high waves

Fever: Ø

Worse: Toward evening; warm or stuffy room; cold wind; getting feet wet

Better: Fresh air; in cold rain; outdoors; cool surroundings

Generalities: Burning pains; pains alternating from left to right

Anas Barbarae
(ann-ass bar-bar-ay)

Anas Barbarae, the best selling flu remedy in France, is marketed as Oscillococcinum by Boiron pharmacy in the US. In France, it has a 50% market share of all influenza medicines sold.

Anas Barbarae is made from the heart and liver of wild waterfowl; the ducks that incubate the flu virus become the instrument of its cure.

Ossi, as it's called, is sometimes not as useful as finding the specific remedy, but it's a good first choice when you feel as though you are coming down with the flu. As a previous chapter shows, many studies have shown it to be helpful. Dana Ullman says it can also be used to treat the common cold.

It works best when taken within the first 48 hours of symptoms. Obviously, it's also a good choice when you are too rushed to sit down and figure out the right remedy. Remember that the difference between a cold and flu is probably body aches, so take it when you start to hurt.

It is similar but not identical to Influenzinum, which is a remedy made from a different virus. I have experienced cases where Ossi didn't work but Influenzinum did, and vice versa.

❖ ❖ ❖ ❖ ❖

The symptoms of Anas Barbarae in the literature are few, but here they are:
✓ Flu remedy for the first onset of flu
✓ Flu remedy for when you are too rushed to find a specific remedy or are uncertain as to the specific remedy

❖ ❖ ❖ ❖ ❖

Other symptoms of Anas Barbarae are:

Cause: Ø

Mind: Fear of contagious disease

Head: Throbbing headache

Face: Ø

Eyes: Tearing

Nose: Stuffed nose with clear discharge, followed by thick discharge

Mouth and Tongue: Ø

Throat: Sore Throat (general)

Larynx: Hoarseness

Neck and Back: Stiff Neck and Back

Chest: Ø

Cough: Cough with thick mucus; Cough (general)

Extremities: Muscle Pain

Stomach: Ø

Food: Ø

Sleep: Ø

Fever: Fever (general); fever of 101°F or above

Worse: Eating milk and eggs

Better: Heat, rest

Generals: Body Aches

Arsenicum Album
(are-sen-i-cum al-bum)

Years ago, the European ladies would powder their faces with arsenic powder to make their complexions white. The arsenic powder gradually seeped through their skin, often making them ill. Unfortunately, it also seeped into their chemistry and left its mark on many of us still. Arsenicum Album remains a very common remedy, both for colds and flu as well as a constitutional, deep acting remedy for those who need it.

All of us have been sick with a bone-chilling cold; we've got the heat turned up to "high," we're in a hot bath several times a day, we're wrapped up in a terry cloth bathrobe, slippers, and blankets, and we can't get warm. There are other remedies that have the symptom of being chilly—such as Nux Vomica—but if you don't fit the Nux Vomica profile, then Arsenicum might be a good choice.

Although all sorts of people might need Arsenicum Album for a cold, Arsenicum Album is famous for treating people who are very tidy or fastidious, almost to a fault. One woman of my acquaintance, who I suspected was an Arsenicum case, not only rubber banded different felt-tip markers by color—which would be usual—but insisted in placing them in the box in a certain order: yellow, pink, red, green, blue. Now, that's Arsenicum! If you tend to be the type of person who alphabetizes his bookcases and sorts things in the medicine cabinet by illness or brand name, you might give Arsenicum a try.

Arsenicum is a good remedy for those who take cold frequently and is also a major hay fever and allergy remedy. Arsenicum is known for treating ailments that are worse in open air and seasonal allergies.

But where Arsenicum is most valuable is as a remedy for stomach flu and food poisoning. It's the first pick for homeopaths when there is vomiting or diarrhea, and especially the two together; when you are actually vomiting and sitting on the toilet at the same time. It's also good for burning diarrhea and stomach upset from eating fruit, vegetables, acid foods, or imbibing too much alcohol. In this case, you would want to take a low dose after each bowel movement or attack of vomiting. Arsenicum also works for mild cases of food poisoning where medical intervention is not necessary. Also, think of Arsenicum when you have dehydration due to fever or diarrhea.

For all these reasons, Arsenicum is a very good choice to take with you when you travel.

Consider Arsenicum when illnesses seem to have some periodicity, such as a fever rising every three hours, waking at the same time each night, recurring colds that happen around the same time every other month, or cold symptoms that recur every week, two weeks, or three weeks.

Think of Arsenicum when you are not sure if you have a cold or hay fever, as Arsenicum and Allium Cepa are major hay fever remedies.

Sulphur, Calcarea Carbonica, and Arsenicum are useful in treating chronic colds where the immune system has broken down.

◈ ◈ ◈ ◈ ◈

Arsenicum has many symptoms, but look for these when you are trying to treat a cold or flu:

✓ High Strung; everything seems too strong and too loud
✓ Extremely chilly, can't get warm
✓ Sufferer may be extremely tidy or neat
✓ Stomach flu or food poisoning
✓ Worse outdoors in open air
✓ Worries about health, death
✓ Congestion usually travels down: Nose → Larynx → Trachea → Chest. Once the cold gets down to the chest, it usually requires a different remedy.
✓ Colds recur with periodicity: same time every year, every month, etc.

◈ ◈ ◈ ◈ ◈

Other symptoms of needing Arsenicum are:

Cause: Grief; fright; swimming in seawater; tobacco smoke; chill in water

Mind: Restless, anxious; and irritable; anxious about health, death, germs, contagion; being left alone; despair of never recovering; hopeless; fearful of anything going wrong; fearful of germs; fearfulness worse at night

Head: Although prefers heat, may prefer cold head; vertigo in the evening or on shutting eyes

Face: Ø

Eyes: Red, with swelling of lids or below the eyes; tears may burn; may be light sensitive

Ears: May have discharge that is thin, burning, or offensive smelling; very sensitive to background noise or of children playing; ears may ring or patient hears bells

Nose: Frequent painful sneezing; discharge from nostrils that burns nose and the upper lip; sneezes with change in temperature; cold begins in the nose and goes down to the throat; thin watery discharge and stuffed up at the same time; tickles in one spot; sneezes a lot and gets no relief from the sneezing; old chronic nasal stuffiness; may be sensitive to odors

Mouth and Tongue: Dry mouth; loss of taste; may have mouth ulcers; tongue bright red or white; creases in tongue

Throat: Hard to cough up mucus in larynx; swallowing difficult; tongue bright red or white; creases in tongue
Larynx: Hoarseness and burning pain

Neck and Back: Ø

Chest: Burning in chest; wheezing; darting pain in upper third of right lung; short of breath; air passages feel constricted

Cough: Worse at night with wheezing respiration; dry cough is worse from drinking and being out of doors; wheezing cough with frothy or bloody expectoration; air passages feel constricted; dry hacking cough

Extremities: Leg cramps

Stomach: Severe nausea, retching, vomiting; vomits immediately eating; (unlike Phosphorus, which vomits water after it becomes warm in the stomach); feels like a stone in stomach; frequent belching

Food: Food tastes bitter; aversion to meat and butter; dislikes smell and sight of food; appetite poor; desires milk, sweets, fat, vinegar, and pickles or other sour foods, but aversion to fat just as likely; prefers warm over cold drinks; gulps hot fluids or sips small amounts; cannot tolerate milk, wheat, and sugar, coffee, ice cream, cold drinks, certain nuts or seafood; alcoholic drinks produce hay fever symptoms

Sleep: Sleep unrefreshing; lies on back with hand under head; wakes at 1:00 in the morning; drowsy by day but restless or agitated at night

Fever: Highest temperature between midnight and 3:00 in the morning; fever of rapid onset with anxiety and restlessness; chills alternate with burning heat

Worse: Drafts; cold food and drinks; cold or wet weather; outdoors in open air; just before and after midnight; after 1:00 in the morning (some say between midnight and 2:00 or 3:00 in the morning); indoor drafts, lying with raised head; lying on right side; light; movement; noise; eating and drinking

Better: Heat, outdoors (even though the nose is stopped up); warm drinks; after eating vegetables; warm food and drink

Generals: Quick movements; fidgety; chills alternate with burning heat; feels intensely hot with fever or intensely cold with chills; skin feels hot (but he feels cold inside); takes cold a lot and sneezes at every change of weather; may be restless or anxious; burning pains in head, back, and extremities; profound weakness; colds that are worse from asthma; sensation of ice or boiling water in veins; restless; achy; skin pale, cold, clammy; chilly, sensitive to drafts

Belladonna
(bell-a-donna)

It is said that Hahnemann treated a little girl for swelling of the finger joints with Belladonna. After a scarlet fever epidemic, Hahnemann noted that the same little girl was the only member of her family not to come down with the dreaded disease. He suspected that the child might have been made resistant to scarlet fever because of the previous Belladonna dose and went on to explore the effect of Belladonna on one of the major diseases of the 19th century. It proved so effective that in 1838 the Prussian Government ordered minute doses of Belladonna to be given to the people as a prophylactic for the disease.

Belladonna is useful in treating the dry sore throat, the red rash, the dilated pupils, and the delirium of scarlet fever, as well as treating the more common Belladonna cold.

Belladonna is native to Greece and Italy, and is a deadly poison in its crude state. Interestingly enough, it is not at all poisonous to goats and rabbits and not as poisonous to any other carnivores except man.

Every beginner in homeopathy knows to associate Belladonna with the symptoms of "hot, dry, sudden, and violent." This is simple to remember: the Belladonna cold often is accompanied by high fever; the person's skin is often dry; and although the fever is high, he has no desire to drink. Belladonna illnesses tend to come on strongly and suddenly and leave quickly.

Despite the violent nature of most Belladonna illnesses, it has been reported that a child with a Belladonna illness may run a high fever but play as though she is not ill.

Belladonna is seldom used for the cold that has taken several days to start, such as one beginning with an achy feeling, progressing to a slight sniffle, developing a nagging dull headache and after that, a tickling throat. Look to another remedy most of the time if the cold has had that kind of slow onset. Belladonna is a lifesaver when it comes to the middle of the night, terribly ill, high-fever-on-the-weekend cold.

Belladonna is a short-term remedy and acts for only up to seven days. It can be repeated in 30C doses as necessary.

◈ ◈ ◈ ◈ ◈

Look for these primary symptoms when you are thinking of Belladonna:
   ✓ Cold with severe headache
   ✓ Dry cold without much nasal discharge
   ✓ Hot, dry, sudden, violent beginning
   ✓ Patient's skin may be red.
   ✓ Pupils dilated
   ✓ One of the first to consider in children's earaches and ear infections
   ✓ Dry red throat worse on the right side
   ✓ Fever with no thirst
   ✓ Cold starts with a nasal discharge, discharge goes away and is replaced by throbbing headache

◈ ◈ ◈ ◈ ◈

Other symptoms of Belladonna include:

Cause: May be caused by exposure to cold air, even as slight as after a hair cut; wet wind

Mind: Nervous anxiety; restlessness

Head: Fullness and pain in forehead, temples, and back of the head; congestive headache; headache is better from wrapping the head tightly; right-sided headache; headache throbs with movement; hot head with cold extremities; dry head without much perspiration; strong pulse of arteries in head; vertigo that makes patient fall to left side or backwards

Face: Flushed face with reddened lips; red face

Eyes: Burning or glassy eyes; dilated pupils; vision may be distorted; twitching in lids; squinting

Ears: Earache, especially in right ear; pus from ears; hearing may either be super acute or dull and noises may reverberate

Nose: Nosebleeds, swelling and redness of nose; reddened nasal membranes; perhaps with hot blood; frequent sneezing; acute sense of smell and may be aware of foul odor in nose; nostril discharge stops and is replaced by throbbing headache and high fever; scanty discharge

Mouth and Tongue: Tongue red at the edge or tip; sore tongue; reddened lips and gums; hot, dry mouth and tongue with an aversion to water

Throat: Feels constricted, dry, red, very painful; worse right side; constriction of throat; stinging pain; throbbing carotid arteries; swelling in the glands of the neck; hard to swallow but wants to keep swallowing, despite the pain; tonsils swollen and/or ulcerated

Larynx: Sudden hoarseness, soreness of larynx; dry larynx; severe laryngitis

Neck and Back: Painful swelling and stiffness of neck and nape of neck

Chest: Snoring breathing; short of breath

Cough: Dry, tearing cough that scrapes throat; sudden cough; cough as if speck in larynx; short croupy or dry cough; tickling, or wet cough with lots of mucus; cough worse when talking or at night; barking or whooping cough

Extremities: Hot head with cold extremities; stinging and burning pains; shooting pains

Stomach: Cramping pains in stomach; good for some cases of nausea and vomiting when other symptoms agree; cramping pain of the stomach extending to the back; stomach cramps are better bending backwards or bending forwards; clutching sensations around the belly button; spasms of the stomach with empty retching

Food: May be either thirstless or have great thirst for cold water; may crave lemonade

Sleep: Scary and violent dreams; moans and groans

Fever: Fevers come on suddenly and tend to be high (above 103°F); starts and jumps during fever; hallucinations during fever; skin is hot to the touch; fevers worse at night; the person may see ghosts, insects, and black animals; the fevers may be accompanied by convulsions or during teething

Worse: Light; jarring the bed; noise; cold wind and drafts; afternoon; lying down; on right side; at night; movement; drinking, stooping, and bending forward; light and sun; worse from pressure and cool surroundings; at 3:00-4:00 in the afternoon, but fever peaks at 9:00 in the evening and 8:00 in the morning

Better: Warmth, standing or sitting upright in a dark room; warm compresses; lying in a dark

place; not moving in a warm room, bending
the head backwards

Generalities: Nervousness; delirium; acute senses;
sensitive to noise or light; flushing and
throbbing symptoms; the child may act in a
violent manner, or bite people; sensitive to
cold and drafts; dry skin but sweats on
covered parts; skin so hot it radiates heat;
right sided symptoms

Bryonia
(bry-oh-nee-uh)

Homeopaths call Bryonia "grumpy bear" because the people who need Bryonia are like hibernating bears: they don't want to be disturbed, they don't want to move, they are better lying still, and they tend to be irritable.

Bryonia has all these characteristics, but as a cold and flu remedy it is invaluable in bringing up mucus in coughs when the cough is loose and the person is having trouble bringing up phlegm.

Bryonia is similar to Arsenicum in that colds begin in the nose, then go down into the throat and larynx, leading to hoarseness and bronchitis.

One important characteristic of Bryonia is that patients are always better when they're still. The only time Bryonia is driven to restlessness is when they are in extreme pain. Quite often, they will be happier lying on a hard surface. Children will often want to lie on the floor.

Like Belladonna patients, they may not want to drink. However, this is different from Belladonna. Belladonna is truly thirstless, and therefore doesn't drink. Bryonia may be thirsty, but does not want to get up and drink something because they really don't want to move. When they do rouse themselves to drink, they drink great quantities at one time.

Bryonia colds and flu come on slowly, over the course of several days of feeling out of sorts. Even fevers tend to be slow in coming and slow to build.

◈ ◈ ◈ ◈ ◈

Look for these symptoms when treating Bryonia colds and flu:

✓ Colds that begin in the nose and the symptoms travel down
✓ Irritable
✓ Thirsty for cold drinks, which they gulp
✓ Wants to lie still and be left alone
✓ Chest has fluid that is hard to cough up
✓ Dry Cough
✓ Coughing with one hand on chest and the other on the head

❖ ❖ ❖ ❖ ❖

Other symptoms of Bryonia include:

Cause: Anger; fright; resentment; embarrassment; weather change from cold to warm

Mind: Anxiety; worried about business, and wants to go home; sympathy makes them feel worse

Head: Severe headache (like Belladonna); bursting, splitting headache; headache is worse from noise, movement, light; stooping; shooting and achyness in forehead; pain in head when coughing; vertigo only when stooping; pain in forehead; the less the nasal discharge the worse the headache

Face: Swollen

Eyes: Pain in eyes when moving them; conjunctivitis; sunlight makes eyes tear; pupils dilated but lack the glint and stare of Belladonna

Ears: Roaring and buzzing in ears; pain in ears; ears feel stopped up

Nose: Mucus membranes dry and stuffy; runny nose with pain in forehead; crusty discharge from nose; swelling of nose; blocked nose

Mouth and Tongue: Tongue coated white, yellow, or brown; lips dry, cracked, bleeding; blisters on edge of tongue; dry mouth, tongue, throat

Throat: Worse in open air; difficult to swallow

Larynx: Mucus in the larynx that is hard to remove; hoarseness

Neck and Back: painful stiffness in the back of the neck; neck, back, and nape of neck sore and better with heat, contrary to the rest of Bryonia symptoms that are better from cold

Chest: Stitches in chest; pressure in chest; hard to take a deep breath

Cough: Hard and dry cough worse at night, or tenacious mucus hard to dislodge; acute bronchitis; chest hurts when coughing; cough worse after eating and drinking, talking, laughing, and smoking; cough worse after taking a deep breath; presses hand to the sternum when coughing

Extremities: Arms and hands painful and weary; pains in limbs

Stomach: A good remedy for summer diarrhea; good for nausea and vomiting with yawning and feeling of faintness

Food: Loss of appetite; food tasteless or too sweet; desires wine, acid drinks, coffee; excessive thirst followed by long drink of cold water

Sleep: Sleepy during day; confused dreams; dreams of daily business; nightmares; sleep delayed at night and unrefreshing; starts awake with fright

Fever: Chilly in the evening, mostly on one side of the body; shivering

Worse: Movement; warm room or being warmly wrapped up

Better: Cold food and drink; cold room; open air

Generalities: Wants to lie still; pain better from pressure; tearing pains; profuse sweats around 2:00 in the morning; sweat has sour smell

Calcarea Carbonica
(cal-care-ree-a car-bon-i-ca)

Look in any homeopathy textbook under Calcarea Carbonica and you will find a picture of a fat, fair-skinned woman, flabby, usually blond and blue eyed, and if it is possible for somebody to look lazy, or at least exhausted, she will look it.

Don't let this stereotype get in your way when you are thinking of remedies for a cold. If Calcarea is not a major cold and flu remedy, it is a least a strong minor one, important in certain cold and flu cases.

Calcarea is a good remedy to think of when there are frequent colds, or where the person does not feel sick but there is a constant, chronic nasal discharge. Calcarea tends to be a chilly remedy; however, the chilliness of Calcarea is one that can be amended by clothing and being in a warm room, whereas Arsenicum cannot be warmed up, because the chill is deeply interior.

Calcarea is known for colds with swollen glands, colds when the patient sweats profusely, especially around the head, and colds accompanied by enlarged tonsils. These three symptoms are a tip-off that Calcarea will be helpful.

As I mentioned in the Arsenicum Album chapter, Calcarea is of use in chronic colds where the immune system has partially broken down.

Some of the major ways to distinguish between a Calcarea cold and another type of cold are the food cravings, aversions, and aggravations. Calcarea is especially marked by strong symptoms in these areas. Of particular note, besides those below, is a marked fondness for eggs. A cold accompanied by a craving for eggs is a sign that Calcarea would be indicated.

◈ ◈ ◈ ◈ ◈

These are the major symptoms of Calcarea:
✓ Recurrent tonsillitis
✓ Painless hoarseness
✓ Colds with swollen glands, especially around the neck
✓ Colds with sweating, especially around the head

◈ ◈ ◈ ◈ ◈

Other symptoms of a Calcarea Carbonica cold include:

Cause: Taking on too much responsibility; exposure to cold water or cold wet weather; sweats with exertion followed by chill or headache; cough may start after exhaustion or fright; drinking alcohol

Mind: Worried about safety, security, home; independent nature; weak memory; afraid of flying, heights, or noise

Head: Feeling of weight on the top of head; headache with cold hands and feet; vertigo on ascending or turning head; head hot with pale face; icy chilliness of head, especially on the right side; headache above right eye, pain extending downward to the nose; throbbing headache; headache is worse stooping; vertigo worse night or early morning

Face: Hot with pale face; puffy face

Eyes: Pressure; burning, stinging in eyes; eyes sensitive to light; itchy eyelids

Ears: Fluid in middle ear; thick yellow discharge; pain or crackling in ears

Nose: Nose congestion lingers; thick yellow nasal discharge; yellow crusts on the outside of nose; nose clogs during the night; nostrils sore; nosebleeds; sneezing with pain in head and nape of neck; inside of nose irritated; sense of smell either acute or dull

Mouth and Tongue: Unpleasant taste in mouth; ulcers in mouth; dry tongue and mouth; lips cracked; tip of tongue feels scalded

Throat: Swelling of tonsils; stitches on swallowing; difficulty swallowing; throat feels constricted

Larynx: Ulcers or lots of mucus in larynx

Neck and Back: Hard, painful swelling of glands in neck; burning or stinging pain in lymph nodes; pain in small of back

Chest: Chest sensitive to pressure; pain after exposure to wet weather; slightest physical effort causes them to be short of breath, especially going upstairs

Cough: Tickling cough worse at night or lying down; cough worse going upstairs; may cough up thick, yellow, sweet tasting mucus

Extremities: Calf, foot, thigh pains or cramps; pain in joints in cold damp weather; cold feet but hot head; joint swelling; tearing in muscles; pain in joints of hip, knees, and feet; legs go to sleep when sitting

Stomach: Frequent sour belching; sour vomiting, diarrhea that is worse in the afternoon; other stomach upset is worse morning, night, and after a meal

Food: Thirst for cold drinks, especially at night; craves eggs, sweets, sour foods, salty food, starches, ice cream, milk, and salt; aversion to meat, boiled foods, and hot foods; wine and milk disagrees

Sleep: Drowsy during the day and early evening; talks or groans in sleep; dreams frequent, vivid, anxious, frightful; dreams of sick or dead people

Fever: Sweats with fever, especially in bed at night; tends to sweat on head, neck, and chest

Worse: Cold damp weather; mental and physical exertion; cold water; cold wet weather; during full moon; anxiety

Generals: Chilly; perspires in sleep; sensitive to cold, especially around ears and neck; takes cold at every change of weather; gets chilled at 2:00 in the afternoon; chill can begin in stomach; skin moist and perspires around the neck, head, and upper body; can be lethargic and passive; prefers loose clothing, especially dislikes tight belts or waistbands; fatigue from the least exhaustion; sweat smells sour

Eupatorium Perfoliatum
(you-pat-tor-ree-um per-foe-lee-ay-tum)

Eupatorium Perfoliatum is a rather uncommon influenza remedy, but when you have the symptoms, and you find relief from Eupatorium, it's a lifesaver.

The major symptom of needing Eupatorium is that you have bone pain (not muscle pain, as in Gelsemium or Bryonia) with severe chilliness. Oddly enough, the chills begin or are worse between 7:00 and 9:00 in the morning, which is an unusual time for an aggravation. The fever is also remarkable in that quite often the person is not thirsty, although they may also be thirstless during the chill phase and then thirsty after the chills have passed.

❖ ❖ ❖ ❖ ❖

The keynote symptoms of needing Eupatorium Perfoliatum are the following:
- ✓ Intense aching limbs and back, bones feel broken
- ✓ Chills with shivering
- ✓ Chills worse between 7:00 and 9:00 in the morning.

❖ ❖ ❖ ❖ ❖

Other symptoms of needing Eupatorium are:

Cause: Ø

Mind: Sadness; restlessness; anxiety; listlessness

Head: Stuffy head feels like it will burst; headache, especially left sided headache with dizziness; headache begins in the morning and gets progressively worse in the afternoon and evening; headache when chilled; headache worse from sweat.

Face: Ø

Eyes: Eyeballs sore; aversion to light

Ears: Ø

Nose: Much sneezing with watery nasal discharge

Mouth and Tongue: Tongue white, corners of mouth sore

Throat: Ø

Larynx: Hoarseness, which is worse in the morning

Neck and Back: Throbbing pain in nape of neck; aching pains in back; weight and heaviness in back; sore back

Chest: Pain in chest when taking a deep breath

Cough: Barking cough with sore chest; cough worse between 2:00 and 4:00 in the morning

Extremities: Aching in arms, wrists, and legs; muscles are sore to the touch, as if beaten; wrists hurt as if broken

Stomach: May vomit bile; increased thirst after chills; stomach pains after eating; nausea from smell of food or after eating or drinking

Food: Craves cold drinks, large quantities of cold water, and ice cream

Sleep: Can't sleep on left side; lies with head high

Fever: Shaking chills; chills preceded by thirst; violent spasms, especially in the morning; fever can go into the chest or to liver to produce jaundice; fever peaks every third day; trembling and nausea from motion during fever; fever helped by sleep

Worse: Cold air; movement; lying on back; chills worse 7:00-9:00 in the morning

Better: Kneeling with face towards pillow or on hands and knees

Generals: Can't move because of pain; sits with hands flat on knees, shoulders raised to support chest/breathing; restless but tries to stay still because movement hurts; similar to Bryonia except bones ache; intolerance of tight clothing

Euphrasia Officinalis
(you-phrase-zha oh-fish-shun-nal-iss)

Several years ago I was living in New York. I didn't really *want* to be in New York, but through a twist of fate I was there, working three jobs—one as Associate Dean of Admissions for St. John's University, one taking care of a friend's elderly parents, and one at the Raindew Department Store up the street. I had heard the phrase "so busy I feel like I'm going to meet myself coming the other way" but I didn't really know what that meant until that year.

My friend with the elderly parents had three dogs and one bed, and when she was out of town I found myself in bed with a huge greyhound, a Doberman, and a small dog of the furry but unknown breed. One morning I woke up with one eye swollen almost shut. Was it an allergy to dog hair? Had I slept with that eye pressed against the pillow?

Dr. Bonnie immediately went to the medicine chest and pulled out a bottle. "This will fix you up," she said, and by the time I grabbed the Long Island Railway that took me back for another day at St. John's, my eye was almost OK.

It turned out the stuff in the little bottle was Euphrasia Officinalis, a plant tincture made from the eyebright plant. Euphrasia isn't used a lot for colds and flu, but if the symptoms fit, it's invaluable. Think of it also for hay fever and seasonal allergies.

◇ ◇ ◇ ◇ ◇

Primary symptoms of Euphrasia Officinalis include:
✓ Burning Tears
✓ Burning swelling of eyelids
✓ A Euphrasia cold will move into the larynx in one or two days and become a hard cough with hoarseness.
✓ Eye symptoms worse outdoors

◈ ◈ ◈ ◈ ◈

Other symptoms of Euphrasia Officinalis include:

Cause: Hay fever

Mind: Does not like to talk; confusion

Head: Shooting pain in temples and forehead; bursting headache with dazzling in front of eyes; stuffy headache with lots of nasal discharge

Face: Cheeks red

Eyes: Sticky mucus on the cornea; tears burn; conjunctivitis; eyes inflamed with profuse tears; dryness and pressure in eyes; eyes light sensitive; acrid and thick discharge from the eyes; eyes ache; eyes tear in cold and windy weather; eyes are worse in open air

Ears: Eardrum pain

Nose: Bland nasal discharge; watery mucus; bloody discharge from nose; nosebleed; nose stopped up at night

Mouth and Tongue: Ø

Throat: Gags when clearing throat in the morning

Larynx: Hoarse in the morning; irritated larynx; phlegm in the larynx; hawks up mucus

Neck and Back: Ø

Chest: Short of breath

Cough: Worse daytime; cough better lying down, but nasal discharge worse; wet cough with profuse phlegm; no cough at night

Extremities: Numbness; painless swelling of fingers and hands; shooting pains in legs or thighs

Stomach: Ø

Food: Ø

Sleep: Ø

Fever: Chill in the morning; sweats at night; fever predominated by chills

Worse: Nasal discharge worse at night; stuffiness worse in the morning; indoors; in warmth; in light; eye symptoms are worse in open air; lying down; at night; windy weather

Better: Ø

Generalities: Cold begins in nose and moves to larynx; fatigue from tired eyes during the day; can't get warm; perspires on upper body only

Ferrum Phosphoricum
(fair-um fos-for-i-come)

Not all colds start violently and suddenly. Some colds start slowly, gradually, with the feeling that you are coming down with something, but it hasn't hit yet. You may spend several days feeling out of sorts and knowing you are about to get a cold but symptoms are still minimal. You have the feeling that you might be able to cut this cold off at the pass if you knew what to do for it. Ferrum Phosphoricum fits this profile.

Ferrum Phos is also useful for the early stage of a cold when the primary symptoms you have are lethargy and a slight fever. Not that Ferrum Phos will not help full-blown cases of cold and flu, because it will—but the main reason you will use Ferrum Phos is to ward off a cold with few symptoms.

One writer suggests that Ferrum Phosphoricum ailments come on faster than Gelsemium but slower than Aconite and Belladonna. It's also not as wet as Bryonia; not as weary as Gelsemium; not as intense as Aconite or Belladonna.

I have not generally listed pulse symptoms in this book, but if you know how to take a pulse, the pulse of Ferrum Phos is noted for being weak and rapid.

❖ ❖ ❖ ❖ ❖

Keynote symptoms of Ferrum Phos include:
✓ Early stages of a cold with few symptoms
✓ Recurrent fever with no symptoms
✓ Colds with nosebleeds of bright red blood

❖ ❖ ❖ ❖ ❖

Other symptoms of a Ferrum Phos cold are:

Cause: Overexertion

Mind: Irritable; talkative; mirthful; forgetful; depression; unable to concentrate; memory impaired

Head: Headache which is better from cold applications; dull headache is worse 5:00 in the afternoon; throbbing in forehead and temples; sharp pain going from back to front of head when stooping; vomiting from pain of headache

Face: Pale face that flushes easily; red face; facial pain

Eyes: Red, feels like sand in eyes; conjunctivitis; light sensitive; inside of lids feel dry and rough; sties on lids

Ears: Earache, especially first stage of ear infection; ringing and buzzing

Nose: First stage of stuffiness; nosebleeds with bright red blood; or blood in nasal discharge; discharge at night

Mouth and Tongue: Dry lips; mouth hot

Throat: Tonsils red and swollen; throat hurts more when swallowing empty; feeling of lump on swallowing; dry and red throat, palate, and tonsils; mucus in throat

Larynx: Irritation or tickling in windpipe; laryngitis

Neck and Back: Stiff neck and back; "crick" in neck and back; shoulder pain; painful swelling of parotid glands

Chest: Breathing oppressed, short, panting; retching and vomiting with cough; dry hacking cough with chest pain; cough better at night; stitching pain breathing in; dry cough; cough worse in cold air; short, painful cough; coughs when deep breathing

Stomach: Vomiting of undigested food; stomach bloated and heavy; intolerance of tight clothes; vomiting at irregular times; pains worse after eating

Food: Poor appetite; craves sour foods like pickles and vinegar; aversion to meat and milk; desires cold drinks

Extremities: Burning soreness of muscles; extremities cold but rest of body hot; joints puffy

Sleep: Drowsy, restless, sleep with anxious dreams; dreams of quarreling that lead to happy conversations with other people

Fever: Chills around 1:00 in the afternoon; fever with no other symptoms

Worse: Night; 4:00-6:00 in the morning; motion; lying right side; open air; sensitive to cold and worse from cold; walking; worse lying in bed and worse from rest; worse eating; physical exertion; cold drinks; heat, near the sea at night; loud noises

Better: Gentle exercise; cold cloth or ice pack; gentle motion; washing face

Generals: Weakness, wants to lie down; diarrhea with fever; stools green or watery; retching at stool; diarrhea worse from midnight to morning

Gelsemium Sempervirens
(gel-sem-me-um sem-per-vy-rens)

If there is one flu remedy that comes to the minds of most homeopaths, it would be Gelsemium Sempervirens, one of the most common of influenza remedies. People needing Gelsemium are extremely weak and feel heavy. The people who respond well to Gelsemium are those who are so weak they can barely get out of bed.

There are a lot of flu remedies that fit people who want to avoid movement, and it's probably not a good idea to use weariness in finding symptoms to treat flu. Anybody with the flu doesn't want to move, but the weakness of Gelsemium tends to be a true weakness, in that they do not move because they are too weak to move, not simply because they don't want to.

Another indicator of Gelsemium is that the flu symptoms seem to hang on and on. If you have someone who can't seem to get over the flu, think of following up the case with Gelsemium.

Gelsemium is also like Ferrum Phos in that it fits someone who is "not well, not ill." When something is wrong, you don't feel well, but you are not sick enough to go to bed or even do much of anything about it.

Gelsemium colds and tend to come on slowly. The only exception is the headache symptom, which may come on very quickly.

One way to differentiate between Gelsemium and Aconite is that the Gelsemium cold comes on a few days after exposure; Aconite comes on in a few hours. Remember that you have to give Aconite soon after the cold begins or it will not be effective. So, if you are torn between the two remedies, give Aconite first.

Another peculiar symptom of Gelsemium is that sufferers are better after they urinate; urination gives them a great sense of relief.

❖ ❖ ❖ ❖ ❖

Keynote symptoms of Gelsemium are:
✓ Flu with extreme weakness
✓ Patient feels too heavy to move
✓ Flu symptoms seem to hang on and on
✓ Patient feels better after they urinate

❖ ❖ ❖ ❖ ❖

Other symptoms of Gelsemium are:

Cause: Summer colds; cold and dry weather; constant excitement or fear; warm moist weather; change of weather; fright; shock; embarrassment; colds and fevers of mild winters

Mind: Dull and listless; dizziness; drowsy; mental apathy; wants to be quiet and left alone; cannot follow one idea for a long time; loss of memory; apathy regarding illness; fear of falling; irritable

Head: Violent, pounding pain in back of head; hot head; bursting headache from neck over to the eyes and forehead; headache (with nausea) in right temple, beginning in the morning and increasing during the day; better sleeping or from vomiting; pulsing of carotid arteries; light-headed, which is worse movement and bright light; heavy aching of the head; feels like a band around head

Face: Flushed face; hot and heavy; yellow face

Eyes: Droopy, heavy eyelids; double vision; blurred vision; one pupil dilated, the other

constricted, or both dilated; eyes feel
bruised; aversion or desire for light

Ears: Shooting pain in ears; rushing and roaring in ears;
earache in cold; shooting pain in ears; pain
in ears when swallowing

Nose: Sneezing; fullness at root of nose; sneezing early in
the morning; dry and hot inside nose; stuffy
with watery discharge; nostrils sore;
sneezing followed by tingling and fullness of
nose; profuse watery discharge which
excoriates nostrils

Mouth and Tongue: Unpleasant taste in mouth; furred
trembling tongue; numb, thinly coated,
yellowish tongue, paralyzed tongue;
difficulty swallowing; (especially warm
food); lips dry, hot, tongue coated yellowish-
white; putrid taste and fetid breath; tongue
red, raw, painful, dry; tongue numb and
feels thick

Throat: Itching and tickling of soft palate; tonsillitis; sore
with red tonsils; difficult swallowing with
earache; lump in throat that cannot be
swallowed; throat can't swallow so liquid
comes out nose; weak throat muscles; dry,
rough, burning throat; sensation of heat and
constriction in throat

Larynx: Weak voice; laryngitis

Neck and Back: Dull aching in neck and back; pain in
mastoid

Chest: Slowness in breathing; sore chest; acute
bronchitis; pneumonia after flu

Cough: Dry cough; teasing, tickling cough

Extremities: Muscle pain; loss of power and muscle control; cramps in forearms; cold extremities with hot head and back; limbs tremble; weak, bruised feeling

Stomach: Sensation of emptiness in stomach; pressure of clothing irritates

Food: Thirstless; increased appetite; small amounts of food satisfy

Sleep: Can't get fully asleep; insomnia from exhaustion; dreams of dying

Fever: Shaking; cold hands and feet with fever; chilliness in the morning; or chilliness at same time each day

Worse: In sun, heat, or hot room; humidity; damp weather; tobacco smoke; fog; emotions or excitement; bad news; thinking of ailment; 10:00 in the morning; fatigue every afternoon between 4:00 and 5:00

Better: After profuse urination; stimulants; alcohol; perspiring; bending forward; open air; continued motion; lying still; physical pressure

Generals: Twitching muscles feel cold and tingly; chills with waves of heat along the spine; muscle weakness, diarrhea from emotional excitement or anticipation of ordeal; nervous chills; high fever with cold extremities

Hepar Sulphuris Calcareum
(he-par sulf-fur-iss cal-care-ee-um)

Homeopaths speak of some symptoms as being "strange, rare, and peculiar," (SRP's), which means that they are specific and unusual symptoms that point to one remedy. One of the SRP symptoms associated with Hepar Sulph is a sensation of wind blowing on one part of the body. If you ever have a condition with this symptom, and the other symptoms agree, I say, Go For It!

Hepar Sulphuris Calcareum is known as a great cure for pus conditions, which is why it is included in this book. If you are ever unfortunate enough to have a cold that is so bad you have pus on your tonsils, in your ears, or coating your throat, Hepar Sulph is a good choice.

Hepar Sulph is not a common remedy for colds; however, it does have very specific symptoms for a cold or flu that make it a valuable cold and flu remedy. It is famous for a sensation of having a splinter in the throat. This condition is felt when swallowing or not swallowing. A person needing Hepar Sulph is worse from cold; after getting chilled he is noticeably worse.

Another main symptom of Hepar Sulph is that they are extremely oversensitive in mind and body. He is sensitive emotionally, sensitive to cold, drafts, or changes in temperature, sensitive to everything that he would not notice as much when he is healthy.

◆ ◆ ◆ ◆ ◆

So, in sum, here are the keynote symptoms of Hepar Sulph:
✓ All the symptoms are worse from cold
✓ Pus conditions of the throat, ears, or other part of the body
✓ Sensation of splinter in the throat
✓ Hypersensitivity of the mind and body

◈ ◈ ◈ ◈ ◈

Other symptoms of Hepar Sulph include:

Cause: Cough starts with exposure to cold air; exposure to cold dry weather; dry cold wind

Mind: Irritable; hypersensitive; complains constantly; asks questions; furious over small matters; abusive; sad (especially in evening); poor memory, especially for words and localities

Head: Ringing and pain in head with cough; vertigo in the evening upon moving the head; headache at night; moving the eyes, headache worse from motion and stooping; cold sweat on head at night and from the least exercise

Face: Yellow with blue circles under eyes

Eyes: Painful and difficult movement of eyes; pressure of eyes; sensation of sand in the eyes; sensitive to light; conjunctivitis with sticky discharge

Ears: Ear pain on swallowing; infection with bloody discharge; darting or shooting pain in ears when blowing nose; itching of ears; (inside and external); scabs behind and around ear; boils inside ear canal

Nose: Sinus congestion; first watery discharge, then becomes thick and yellow, or thick and yellow from the beginning; nose swollen and painful; sneezes at least exposure to cold air; or profuse discharge; sense of smell lost or very acute; nasal discharge smells like old cheese

Mouth and Tongue: Tonsillitis; cold sores; mouth ulcers; blisters on lips; increased salivation; crack in the center of lower lip

Throat: Cold starts with itchy, tickling throat; fish bone, splinter, or crumb sensation; hawks up mucus; swallowing difficult; sore throat with ulceration; sensitive tonsils with red glottis

Larynx: Hoarseness from cold dry wind; pain in larynx when swallowing; hoarseness worse from talking or coughing

Neck and Back: Swelling on neck painful to touch; pulsing carotids; shooting pain in shoulder blades and neck

Chest: Rattling of phlegm in chest, especially in sleep; sore chest; short of breath; tenacious mucus in chest

Cough: Cough worse in cold air; coughs from pain in the larynx; worse evening until midnight; worse eating or drinking anything cold; can't bring mucus up; dry loose cough or barking cough; thick yellow mucus; cough loose, rattling cough, sensation of strangling and gagging from cough; coughs when any body part is uncovered; bending the head backward brings relief from the cough

Extremities: Cold perspiration on hands; itchy palms; weak limbs; pains worse in cold weather

Stomach: Alternate nausea and chills; nausea in the morning; pressure in stomach after eating only a little food

Food: Strong thirst; desires vinegar; loss of appetite; desires acid food, spicy, strong-tasting food or alcoholic drinks; aversion to fat

Sleep: Yawning; sleepy; prolonged sleep or sleeplessness, especially sleepless late at night

Fever: Chill in evening; especially from 6:00 to 7:00; alternate chills and heat during the day, with profuse perspiring; chill from the slightest breeze

Worse: Getting cold, undressing; from the least draft, evening until midnight; morning and evening; touch, pressure, motion, cold wind; cold dry weather; exertion

Better: Eating; warm compresses; warm room; heat, bundling up; moist, wet weather (opposite of Gelsemium); hot drinks

Generals: Sensitive to touch, pain, disturbance; hypersensitivity to pain; sweats at night without relief

Influenzinum
(in-flu-en-zee-num)

I came close to not putting this remedy in *Cure That Cold! Fight That Flu!*, because there are few homeopathy books that list it.

I could not find specific symptoms for Influenzinum in any of the books in my bibliography, which is why there are no symptoms listed by body part below, no keynote symptoms, and no symptoms in the Repertory at the end of this book. But I wanted to give it honorable mention.

It is very similar in use to Anas Barbarae. Influenzinum is made from the actual flu virus, and Anas Barbarae is made from the heart and liver of ducks, which carry the flu virus.

There have been occasions when Anas Barbarae did not work for the flu but Influenzinum did, and vice versa. I would suggest that if you pick Anas Barbarae and it doesn't work, and if you are certain what you have is influenza and not a cold, try Influenzinum instead.

Like Anas Barbarae, it's possible to take it weekly in the wintertime to help protect against getting the flu. It's a good remedy to have on hand when you travel, as well.

Kali Bichromicum
(kay-lie by-cro-mick-um)

Every profession has sources of humor. I sometimes wonder just why I ended up in a profession where I had to be intimately involved with many varieties of nasal discharge. I do have days when I think if I have to ask one more person what color his nasal discharge is, I will permanently go off my feed. (That, or jump in my car, change my name, and find a job that is as far away from bodily secretions as I can. . .)

Well, in this case, you've got to think about mucus, because one of the keynotes of Kali Bichromicum is ropy and yellow discharge. This is true for both eye and nasal discharges.

Kali Bichromicum is not usually useful in the first stage of a cold or flu; it is much better for the ripe cold where the secretions have really started and you feel like you're in for a long haul.

◈ ◈ ◈ ◈ ◈

The keynote indications for Kali Bichromicum are few, but here they are:

✓ Sensation of a hair in back of throat, back of left nostril, or tongue (compare with "splinter" in throat for Sulphur)
✓ All discharges are thick, ropy, yellow or yellow-green.
✓ Constantly blowing nose
✓ Pain when sticking out tongue

◈ ◈ ◈ ◈ ◈

Here are more symptoms of Kali Bichromicum:

Cause: Spring and autumn ailments; overindulgence in beer or malt beverages

Mind: Talks in excessive detail; avoids people; listless; aversion to work; weak memory

Head: Headache worse in the morning; headache over eyebrows or pressure on top of head; scalp feels sore; migraine with visual impairment or blindness; headache is worse from light, noise, walking, stooping, and at night and is accompanied by nausea and vomiting; headache may also be worse at 9:00 in the morning; headache is better open air; lightheadedness in the morning on stooping

Face: Pressing pain that feels as though cheekbones and bridge of nose is being pressed; red or pale face

Eyes: Eyelids burn, swell, and itch; heavy eyelids in the morning; eyes water; yellow matter in corners of eyes; feeling of sand in eyes; eyeballs red; eyes sensitive to sunlight

Ears: Stinging pain shooting into head; pain in left ear; pain in ear extends to roof of mouth; hard swelling of left parotid gland; heat and itching in external ears

Nose: Pain at root of nose better by pressure; constantly blowing nose; discharge worse in cold and open air; thick mucus; pressure at sinus and root of nose; nose dry and stopped up; loss of smell; nasal stuffiness worse in warm air, better in cool air; stuffy noses of children, especially fat, chubby babies; discharge greenish yellow; discharge sticks like glue; tough, elastic plugs in nose; tough green

mucus in nose; violent sneezing, worse in
open air; sensation of a hair in left nostril

Mouth and Tongue: Pain when sticking out tongue;
tongue coated brown; tongue red and shiny;
tongue dry, smooth, red and cracked; mouth
dry; lower lip swelled, chapped, and cracked

Throat: Thick postnasal drip with sticky mucus; swollen
throat relieved by cold; tickle in back of
throat; dry and rough throat; pain better
swallowing hot liquid; sharp, shooting pain
left tonsil; ulcers in the throat; tonsils
swollen and inflamed; sensation of plug in
throat not better by swallowing

Larynx: Hoarse voice, worse in evening; wakes 2:00 in
the morning with sensation of choking

Neck and Back: Swollen lymph nodes or parotid gland
(behind jaw) stiff neck when bending
forward; pain in tailbone, worse walking,
worse sitting

Chest: Sensation of pressure and heaviness on chest,
better after rising

Cough: (Not useful in beginning stages of cough.) Later,
brassy cough that is worse in the morning

Extremities: Pains in limbs that change location quickly;
feel bruised; cracking in joints; pain in calf
tendons

Stomach: Sudden nausea; thirsty; loss of appetite;
stomach upset by mild food; heartburn after
meal; heartburn pain may extend to the
back; vomiting after any attempt to eat or
drink; can't bear tight clothing; vomits

bright yellow water; food lies in stomach like heavy stone

Food: Increased thirst; desires cold drinks, beer, and sweets; aversion to meat; meat upsets stomach

Sleep: Rattling breathing during sleep; unrefreshing sleep; wakes at 2:00 in the morning with nausea or headache

Fever: Chills with trembling

Worse: Worse in the morning, especially at 3:00; from alcohol; cold damp weather; 2:00-3:00 in the morning; open air; when snow is melting; worse from touch and stooping

Better: Expectorating fluid; lying in bed; heat; movement

Generals: Pain in small spots; pain moves from place to place; sharp and burning pain

Lycopodium Clavatum
(lie-co-po-dee-um clav-vay-tum)

Lycopodium Clavatum, a remedy made from club moss, is not a very common cold and flu remedy, but it is interesting for its psychological symptoms. People who need Lycopodium Clavatum as remedy for a chronic, long-standing illness tend to equate physical weakness with moral deficiency. They will often not give in to a cold because they see illness as a sign of weakness, yet they are ill longer because they refuse to take care of themselves.

The ailments of Lycopodium Clavatum tend to be right sided or move from right to left. We often see this in the sore throat of a Lycopodium Clavatum cold, where the pain is right-sided at first and then moves to the left, or starts on the left and then spreads to both sides of the throat.

Lycopodium Clavatum colds tend to start in the nose and go down to the chest. This is similar to Arsenicum.

One weird symptom of Lycopodium Clavatum is that the sore throat is better from holding cold water in the mouth, even before the patient swallows.

◈ ◈ ◈ ◈ ◈

So, in sum, these are the important Lycopodium Clavatum symptoms:

✓ Better holding cold water in the mouth
✓ Cold settles in nose and goes to chest
✓ Equates physical weakness with moral deficiency
✓ Right sided sore throat or moves from right to left

◈ ◈ ◈ ◈ ◈

Other symptoms of needing Lycopodium Clavatum are:
Cause: Fear; fright; chagrin; anger; anxiety; wine

Mind: Fearful but can be bossy; afraid to be alone; spells words wrong or uses them in the wrong way; wakes angry or cross; despondent; memory weak; holds grudges; drops letters out of words; in a hurry; lump in throat on emotional occasions

Head: Head pain better in cold weather and with motion; the headache returns when thick yellow discharge returns; headache worse on the top of the head; headache with vertigo; headache worse stooping; headache worse lying down; headache worse between 4:00-8:00 in the evening

Face: Pale face, paler in evening; blue circles around eyes; redness of cheeks; swelling of upper lip

Eyes: Aching in eyes; dry eyes; mucus in eyes; swelling of lids; night blindness

Ears: Thick yellow offensive-smelling ear drainage; tinnitus; eczema; congestion and ulceration of ears; humming and roaring in ear; eczema behind and around ears

Nose: Chronic thick yellow discharge; crusty nasal discharge; fan-like movement of nose; food and drink regurgitated through the nose; nose blocked at night causing the patient to mouth breathe

Mouth and Tongue: Tip of tongue feels scalded; dry mouth with no thirst; tongue coated; blistered tip of tongue

Throat: Swelling and suppuration of tonsils; better swallowing warm fluids; constriction in throat; obstructed swallowing; burning pain in throat

Larynx: Voice weak and dull

Neck and Back: Stiffness left side of neck; swelling of glands

Chest: Wheezing; throbbing, heaviness, and burning in chest; unresolved pneumonia; bronchitis

Cough: Wet cough in the daytime with expectoration and dry cough at night with no expectoration; cough worse between 4:00-6:00 in the evening

Extremities: Stiff elbow and wrist; joint pain; stiff knees; cold feet, or one hot and the other cold

Stomach: Constant nausea, bloated abdomen; bloated after small amount of food; gas and belching; gnawing and burning pain in stomach; rumbling and diarrhea; nausea from motion; especially in the morning

Food: Appetite capricious; loss of appetite; a little food fills up with gas; aggravation from cabbage, peas, milk, pastry, onions, broccoli, and beans; reheated food gives indigestion; craves sugar and sweets; wants hot meals and liquids; aversion to coffee, rye bread, cooked meats or warm foods; either absence of thirst or burning thirst

Sleep: Disturbed and restless sleep; anxious and frightful dreams; restless limbs at night

Fever: Worse between 4:00-8:00 in the evening; sensation of numbness in the hands and feet during fever; nausea and vomiting when chilled; sweats from least exercise

Worse: Tight clothes; overeating; room temperature or cold food and drinks; first waking and 4:00-8:00 in the evening; gets sick from skipped meals; tobacco smoke; cold air; right side; hot air in bed

Better: Loose clothes; movement; cool air; warm drinks; eating; loosening clothes; getting cold; movement

Generals: Symptoms right sided or move from right to left or go from above downwards; dislikes tight clothing on abdomen; chilly; chair or couch feels hard

Mercurius Vivus
(Mur-cure-ree-us viv-us)

In the early days of homeopathy, homeopaths used to make a solution of Mercurius Solobilus, which was the ammonium nitrate of Mercury. A lot of preparation was needed to make this remedy, and later, when it was found that the symptoms it relieved were identical to Mercurius Vivus, homeopaths began to use that instead.

There are several different types of Mercurius, and what I will discuss is the most common form. It's the same as Mercurius Hydrargyrum, or Mercurius Oxydulatus. You'll probably see it most often listed as Mercurius Sol or Mercurius Viv, sometimes as Quicksilver.

Mercurius is valuable for a particular kind of cold. With this type of cold there is a lot of saliva and the mouth is really wet. The patient drools on the pillow and when talking. He has a bitter, metallic taste in his mouth. The tongue is "flabby" and holds the imprint of his teeth. The glands may be swollen and he may sweat profusely.

Many homeopathic researchers believe there is a link between having a lot of amalgam fillings in your mouth and having the Mercurius cold. Mercury is a small component of an amalgam filling, and it is postulated that the mercury is absorbed in minute amounts into the body and this in turn gives people symptoms of mercury poisoning. Remember, in the opening chapters of this book we read how a crude dose of a substance will give symptoms that a minute dose will take away, and that is how this process may work. Opinions vary, however, as to the usefulness of the removal of amalgam fillings and how much they actually affect patient health. It's unproven if these fillings are the source of the Mercurius cold.

One strange, rare, and peculiar symptom of Mercurius Vivus is that patients needing it will sneeze when exposed to direct sunshine.

Mercury is a rather unusual remedy for a cold, but once again, if the symptoms fit, don't be afraid to use it.

❖ ❖ ❖ ❖ ❖

Keynote symptoms of Mercurius are:
   ✓ Ropy, stringy saliva (like Kali Bichromicum)
   ✓ Drools on pillow
   ✓ Pale, swollen, flabby tongue that shows imprint of teeth
   ✓ Gray ulcers on tongue or gums or palate

❖ ❖ ❖ ❖ ❖

Other symptoms of Mercurius Vivus are:

Cause: Fright

Mind: Easily frightened; slow answering questions; restless; forgets names of people, streets, and places; indifferent; angry; suspicious

Head: Cloudiness and dizzy when getting up; heavy aching in head; head is tender to touch and feels as if it is in a vise, and the pain makes the patient nauseated; headache is worse outdoors, sleeping, eating or drinking; head pain when coughing; headache is worse at night and upon waking, better up and moving around; vertigo when lying on back; loss of hair

Face: Pale, yellowish; puffy; flashes of heat in face with ice cold extremities; hot and cold sensations

Eyes: Pressure in the eyes; profuse tears; lids red, swollen; burning, acrid tears; eyes made sore from heat; eyes feel cold; photophobia; eyes red; pupils dilated

Ears: Tearing, shooting pains in the ears; burning discharge; roaring in ears; cold feeling in ear; pus in ear; swelling of right parotid gland (gland in front of or below the ear) with stinging pain

Nose: Ulcers in nose; nostrils raw and sore; nosebleeds with clotted black blood; pain and swelling of nose with greenish or yellow-green discharge; frequent sneezing with clear nose; nose red, swollen, shining; itching in nose; dry stuffiness or fluent discharge

Mouth and Tongue: Tongue red and swollen; tongue feels burnt; breath foul; tongue cracked down upper center; metallic, salty, bad taste in mouth; teeth ache with hot or cold fluids, better rubbing the cheek on that side; lips dry, rough, blackish; scabs or ulcers on lips; tongue wet and coated; ulcers on tongue

Throat: Painful dryness of throat; raw sore throat; mouth filled with saliva; sore throat worse swallowing empty; ulcers in throat or on tonsils; swallowing painful; inability to swallow; liquids go through nostrils; bluish-red swelling of throat

Larynx: Burning and tickling in larynx with hoarseness

Neck and Back: Burning pain at nape and back of neck; swelling of neck glands; neck and lower back sore as from bruise; enlargement of lymph nodes; swelling of salivary glands

Chest: Difficult respiration; short of breath; sensation of dryness in chest; stabbing pain from right lung to back; bronchitis; coughing worse evening and night

Cough: Worse at evening and night; bloody, thick, green expectoration; dry, rough, tickling cough; cough with retching, choking, and vomiting

Extremities: Weakness in limbs; trembling extremities; bone pain, especially at night when warm in bed; joints painful; jerking in arms and fingers; sweaty palms; feet cold and sweaty

Stomach: Nausea with pain in stomach and chest; cramps in stomach after eating only a little; vomiting of mucus; hiccupping after meal

Food: Hungry; thirsty for cold drinks, especially milk and beer; desires wine, alcohol; rye bread has bitter or sweet taste; aversion to butter, meat, fat, cooked food, coffee; bread, butter, sweets aggravate

Sleep: Drowsy in daytime; deep sleep or trouble getting to sleep and wakes too early; dreams of robbers, gunshots, and biting dogs; vivid, terrifying, anxious dreams makes him wake frequently with palpitations and sweating

Fever: Chills early in the morning and when rising; fever comes on after midnight with thirst; debilitating night sweats; chills between diarrhetic stools

Worse: At night; warmth of bed; damp cold; rainy weather; sweat; very cold or very hot weather; autumn

Better: Morning; resting

Generals: Swelling of face; body feels bruised; feels bad in a warm room, but cannot bear cold; extensive sweating with fever but does not make him feel better; offensive sweat; exhaustion after slight exertion; watery diarrhea, or dark brown, yellow, or green stools

Natrum Muriaticum
(nay-trum myur-ee-at-i-come)

Natrum Muriaticum, a remedy made from salt, is a common cold remedy. Unlike the other remedies, where your choice is mostly based on physical symptoms, giving Natrum Muriaticum can be based on emotional symptoms or painful circumstances. In this way it is like Nux Vomica, the use of which can be based on any cold that follows overwork or exhaustion.

Natrum Muriaticum colds tend to follow on the heels of grief, fright, emotional stress, or shock. This is true for both long term and short-term grief. Natrum Mur is useful for the colds or flu that follows death, divorce, or the loss of a job, where the symptoms also agree. There is also a Natrum Mur personality that has a large amount of grief throughout life who, when the patient gets a cold, tends to have a Natrum Muriaticum cold.

People needing Natrum Mur have a tendency to have tears run from their eyes when they laugh. Natrum Mur is also famous for healing fever blisters and mouth ulcers. If someone has a mouth ulcer, look at Nat Mur to see if the rest of the symptoms fit.

Another classic Natrum Mur symptom is a thin, watery nasal discharge. The nose drips like a faucet on the pillow when the patient is asleep or when he bends over.

◈ ◈ ◈ ◈ ◈

So in brief, here are the prominent Natrum Muriaticum symptoms:

✓ Colds and flu after emotional grief, anger, or shock
✓ Watery nasal discharge that drips like from a faucet
✓ Colds with mouth ulcers or fever blisters

✓ Tears with laughter

❖ ❖ ❖ ❖ ❖

Other symptoms of Natrum Muriaticum are:

Cause: Becomes ill after parents' quarrel; grief; death; divorce; loss; rejection; unrequited love; fright; drafts, stress or shock

Mind: Either very depressed or very happy; annoyed by sympathy; desires solitude; consolation makes the patient worse; sensitive; suffers slights and disappointments in silence, but harbors resentment over them

Head: Vertigo with a tendency to fall forward and to the left; bursting headache with cough; headache worse in the morning; headache on forehead or one-sided; headache with pallor, nausea, and vomiting, better lying down, or lying with head high; headache is better after vomiting; headache between 10:00-11:00 in the morning

Face: Yellow or pale face

Eyes: Profuse, watery discharge; sensation of grit in eyes; eyes feel bruised; eyelids heavy; eyes tear when coughing

Ears: Roaring in ears

Nose: Excessive sneezing; inflammation and swelling of nose; either very dry or very runny nose; abnormal quantity of secretion; loss of sense of smell; blisters on sides of nose; sneezes often; profuse discharge, then stopped up or dry; discharge of thick white mucus, like egg white

Mouth and Tongue: Mouth dry; lips dry, cracked, chapped; numbness and tingling of tongue or lips; mouth ulcers; fever blisters; loss of sense of taste

Throat: Feels like a plug in throat when swallowing; frequent hawking of mucus

Larynx: Hoarseness

Neck and Back: Pain in the back, better with firm support; aching, rigidity, painful stiffness in neck; tension in neck

Chest: Pains in chest

Cough: Tickling cough; short chronic cough; bloody mucus, retching and vomiting with cough

Extremities: Palms hot and perspiring; numbness and tingling in fingers; hangnails

Stomach: Feels like lump in stomach after eating; violent hiccups; nausea in the morning

Food: Craves or avoids salt; desires cold drinks; craves cold drinks even when chilled; very thirsty, especially for tea; aversion to bread, slimy food, fats

Sleep: Difficulty falling asleep

Fever: Headache and chill during fever; chill between 9:00 and 11:00 in the morning or 12:00 noon; doesn't recover after fever

Worse: 10:00-11:00 in the morning; sudden noises; music; lying down; getting hot; fresh air; 10:00 to 11:00 in the morning; extremes of temperature; from sleep; lying on the left side; noise; may be either better or worse at seaside; worse touch and pressure

Better: Open air, even though patient caught the cold from a draft; lying down makes vertigo and headache better, but cough is worse; getting out of bed

Generals: Pains like electric shock, with twitching, jerking, and trembling; chill not helped by covering up; urine spurts when coughing; sweats while eating

Nux Vomica
(nucks vom-ik-ka)

Nux Vomica is probably the most common remedy homeopaths dispense. Many homeopaths give Nux Vomica automatically as a first prescription because it will clear the patient of the residues of previous prescription or non-prescription drugs.

Nux Vomica will also treat many illnesses, regardless of type, that come on after overwork or stress. College students who get sick right after finals, accountants right after tax time, mother's colds that come on right after a huge family wedding—all will probably benefit from a dose of Nux Vomica. It's a favorite remedy of mine anytime a child comes down with a cold on December 26th, after two days of being overstimulated, excited, wild and crazy.

It's a really good remedy for people who strive to be the first and the best, ambitious types who don't know when to stop. Nux is especially indicated when the workaholic relies on coffee or other stimulants to keep working. It also fits the party types, who drink, smoke, dance, and don't get enough sleep.

Nux Vomica is especially good for stomach distress arising from overwork. Often when the patient is struck with nausea he says, "If only I could vomit" because they are nauseated and feel that if he could vomit he would get rid of what is making them sick and feel better.

Another use of Nux Vomica is for new babies with sniffles.

Nux Vomica works best if it is taken in the evening at bedtime, not in the morning or after eating.

◈ ◈ ◈ ◈ ◈

So, in summary, these are the primary symptoms of Nux Vomica:

✓ When the illness is a result of taking prescription
drugs
✓ Colds resulting from overwork, exhaustion
✓ Colds of workaholics
✓ Nausea that feels as though it would be better if
the patient could vomit
✓ Newborns with sniffles

❖ ❖ ❖ ❖ ❖

Other symptoms of Nux Vomica include:

Cause: Prolonged mental and emotional stress or
exertion; stimulants; (coffee, medicine);
overindulgence in food and drink; cold and
dry weather; sedentary life; anger; drugs
(prescription and recreational); overwork or
lack of sleep

Mind: Oversensitive, critical, and irritable; sensitive to
noise, movement, pain, and odors; easily
offended; frustrated in little things; tense;
angry; fussy and tidy; resents consolation;
doesn't want to be touched; omission of
words or syllables when writing

Head: Headache worse from not eating (Lycopodium
Clavatum, Arsenicum Album headaches are
better from eating), anger, open air, waking;
occipital or frontal headache; pain on top of
head, as from a nail; cough brings on
headache; heaviness and feeling of pressure
in head; one sided headaches after too much
coffee; vertigo with momentary loss of
consciousness; vertigo after a meal, walking,
being in open air, sneezing, coughing,
stooping; sore scalp and roots of hair

Face: Circles around eyes; pale face, yellowish around
nose and mouth; sweats on face; swelling of

one side of the face; one-sided facial neuralgia (pain running along a nerve) with watery nasal discharge from nostril on the painful side of face; pain spreads to the ear on the painful side

Eyes: Sensitivity to light, especially in the morning; dry eyes; dry, itchy, swelling and redness of lids; pupils either dilated or contracted; black spots in front of eyes

Ears: Itching of the middle ear; frequent swallowing for relief; noises too loud; loud sounds are painful; blockage of Eustachian tube with mucus; mucus in ears; acute pain in ears, especially when swallowing; ringing, roaring, hissing in ears; ears crackling when chewing

Nose: Initially stuffed up and dry, then turning into runny nose; nose itches; tip of nose cold; nose alternates between watery discharge and blocked; colds with blocked nose at night and running during the day; odors, especially perfume and tobacco, irritate or make ill; sneezing fits; nose runs in warm room and stuffed up outdoors; nose better in cold air; nosebleed with clots of dark blood from nose

Mouth and Tongue: Mouth dry; mouth ulcers; bad smell from mouth; tongue coated white; thick or yellow coating; acid, salt, sweet, bitter, metallic taste in mouth; tongue feels thick

Throat: Rough and scraped, raw, sore; tickle or constriction of throat; throat pain worse when not swallowing

Larynx: Pain in larynx with cough; painful hoarseness or roughness of larynx; spasms in larynx, feels like suffocating; sensation of a plug in throat

Neck and Back: Painful stiff neck; backache 3:00-4:00 in the morning; pulling pain as from a bruise; rigidity of nape of neck; swelling of parotid glands; pain in glands when swallowing; bruised pain in small of back

Chest: Shallow respiration; short of breath which is worse at night or in the morning; constricting pain in chest

Cough: Cough with retching; cough ends in retching; sporadic cough with soreness of chest; dry, tearing cough; dry hacking cough

Extremities: Stiff, aching neck; muscle tension; arms and legs go to sleep; rheumatic pains in shoulders and arms; pains in wrists; hands and fingers numb; weakness of limbs; cramps in calves

Stomach: Feeling of weight or swelling in stomach; stomach pain one to one-and-a-half hours after eating; clothes have to be loosened; chronic indigestion; vomiting with much retching, gagging, and straining; gas, heartburn, nausea after eating; shivering after drinking; belching; wants to belch but constriction prevents it; cramps in stomach; acid reflux; nausea worse in the morning; pain in stomach extends to shoulders

Food: Loss of appetite; no hunger; either thirsty or dislikes to drink; tolerates other fatty foods but animal fat disagrees; desires spicy food, fat, coffee, alcohol or milk; meat causes nausea; desires stimulants; hunger but

dislike of food; feeling of fullness after
eating little food

Sleep: Frequent waking at 3:00 in the morning; any noise
disturbs and wakes up; when he wakes up at
3:00 he feels good, can't fall asleep until the
morning, then wakes up feeling wretched;
light sleep; drowsy after lunch or in the
evening

Fever: Fever, when fever is a side effect from drugging;
chills predominate with fever; blue
fingernails; worse uncovered; shivers when
moved

Worse: In the morning; open air; motion; mental
exertion; after midnight; 3:00-4:00 in the
morning; 8:00-9:00 in the evening; anxiety;
getting wet (but better wet weather); eating;
coffee; tobacco smoke; windy weather; cold
food; cold water; wine, touch; cold, dry,
windy weather; open air; stimulants; spicy
food; noise; outdoors; overexertion; light

Better: Wet weather; asthma better outdoors, all else
worse; warmth; firm pressure; sleep; left
alone; in the evening; lying down; after
adequate unbroken sleep; evenings

Generals: Chills alternating with heat; sensitive to the
least draft; pain threshold is low; faints
from odors when ill; tight clothes aggravate;
may do everything rapidly; tense before
thunderstorms; hates sound of wind;
morning diarrhea; inability to turn around
in bed without sitting up; chill and shivering
at slightest movement; constipated with no
desire for bowel movement

Phosphorus
(fos-for-us)

Homeopathic literature is full of descriptions of Phosphorus as a constitutional remedy. Phosphorus is good for a number of complaints, especially when the mental complaints of fearfulness, lack of concentration, or poor memory accompany a cold. The interesting thing about a Phosphorus case is that the patient sometimes doesn't show how sick he is. Being people pleasers, Phosphorus patients love company and act like they feel better when they have someone with them.

In terms of colds and flu, Phosphorus colds often begin in the chest. Phosphorus cures many kinds of coughs, wet or dry. It's very valuable when used on the dry night cough that is worse when lying down.

Those needing Phosphorus can be "faddish" about foods, following one healthy diet after another, one week vegetarian, one week raw foods, one week macrobiotic, and so on.

Please Note: It is very important to remember not to use Phosphorus on a patient if there is any chance the person has tuberculosis. It can make his case worse and cause the tuberculosis to spread. I would not use it if the patient has ever had a positive TB test; in that case, I would use the next indicated remedy.

❖ ❖ ❖ ❖ ❖

Keynote symptoms of Phosphorus are:
✓ Poor concentration
✓ Poor memory
✓ Colds begin in the chest
✓ Dry cough
✓ Gregarious and wants company when sick

❖ ❖ ❖ ❖ ❖

Other symptoms of a Phosphorus cold are:

Cause: Cold after getting haircut; getting a chill to the head

Mind: Needs attention; fearful, including fear of the dark, thunderstorms, spiders, disease, or ghosts; sympathetic; friendly; affectionate; artistic; lack of follow-through; gets angry quickly and is quickly remorseful; apathy alternating with anger

Head: Throbbing headache; sits up and wants cold compresses to head; sneezing and coughing causes pain to the head; hunger precedes and accompanies headache; headache is worse stooping, from a change of temperature, or while eating but better after eating; dizziness, especially in the morning; back of head cold; skin of forehead feels tight

Face: Pale, swollen face

Eyes: Sore to the touch; vision better in the twilight; disturbances of vision; eyes tear and water

Ears: Yellow discharge from ears; deafness with cold in head; difficulty in hearing, especially the human voice; ears burn and throb

Nose: Painful dryness in nose; nose alternately blocked and running; or, one nostril blocked and the other running; streaks of blood when blowing nose; loss of smell; dry scabs in nose; nose red, shiny, sore

Mouth and Tongue: Cracked lips, crack in the center of lower lip; bleeding gums; too much saliva or dryness of mouth; sputum tastes salty, sour, or sweet; tongue coated white

Throat: Dry throat, sneezing causes pain in throat; tonsils and uvula swollen; clears throat frequently

Larynx: Laryngitis without pain; worse in the evening; mucus in larynx

Neck and Back: Swollen glands in neck; stiff neck and back; burning pain in back; spine tender, especially between shoulder blades and small of back; pain in coccyx (tailbone)

Chest: Empty feeling in the chest; cough better in bed; tightness or feeling of weight in chest; noisy or panting respiration; dryness of air passages; chest pain, especially left side; pleurisy, especially of the right lung; pneumonia

Cough: Raspy cough so painful patient tries not to cough; cough worse lying on left side, in open air, when laughing, around strong odors, in cold air, or from talking; dry, tickling, persistent, exhausting cough; cough causes retching or vomiting; cough better from cold drinks; cough first dry, then loose; coughs up yellow phlegm, bright red blood or rusty discharge; mucus when coughed up tastes salty or sweet

Extremities: Limbs weary or stiff; coldness or heat in hands; cramping in limbs; arms, fingers, and hands easily numb

Stomach: Nausea and vomiting due to food poisoning; stomach flu; vomits as soon as drink is warm in stomach; pains in stomach better from cold drinks and food; frequent belching; nausea and empty hunger in the morning

Food: Craves cold drinks, salt, milk, chocolate, ice cream, fish, spicy food, or carbonated drinks; dislikes meat, tea, coffee, beer; desires but more often aversion to fish; too much salt aggravates; hunger between meals; can be "faddish" about foods

Sleep: Sleepy 7:00 in the evening but falls asleep late; wakeful at night, but sleeps in the daytime; anxious, depressing, frightful, or horrible dreams; or dreams of unfinished business

Fever: Shivering; chills with transient heat

Worse: Going from warm to cold and vice versa; in the evening; while fasting; physical and mental exertion; warm food and drinks; change of weather; twilight and evening; before and during a thunderstorm

Better: Lying on the right side; sitting; being with other people; warm applications; open air; sound sleep; massage

Generals: Sensitive to external stimuli; trembling; fidgety; tobacco makes patient nauseated and causes heart palpitations; tendency for watery and painless diarrhea or constipation with hard dark feces; involuntary stool when coughing

Pulsatilla Nigricans
(pul-sa-till-a ny-gri-cans)

Pulsatilla is one the most commonly used cold remedies. It suits the ripe cold, with plenty of nasal discharge that is a thick yellow or green. It is rare that you will give Pulsatilla for the early stages of a cold, but the golden rule of homeopathy is to look at all the symptoms, and, by all means, if Pulsatilla fits, give it.

Pulsatilla is called "the weathercock" because one of the keynote symptoms of Pulsatilla is change. The patient may be of a changeable temperament, or the symptoms may change. The location of body pain may change from place to place; the type of pain may change, from sharp to a dull ache; he may have a scratchy throat one minute, then an hour later, the throat is fine but then he has a headache; several hours later the head is fine but he has ear pain and lassitude. . . and so it goes.

Pulsatilla is a wonderful remedy for ear pain or ear infections, and is one of the first remedies to think of when a young child has an ear infection. Belladonna is also indicated for ear infections, but Pulsatilla ailments do not come on as fast or as violently.

Those needing Pulsatilla are extremely sensitive and impressionable. The patient often "picks up" the vibes of others. If a child's parents say that he is better, then he will be. If the parents worry about him and say he's worse, then he will be.

Like Phosphorus, Pulsatilla wants consolation, and young children will be very clingy, literally so. In adults this is sometimes manifested by the person who is obviously sick but who keeps coming into the family room or will not leave the gathering to go to bed.

◈ ◈ ◈ ◈ ◈

So, the keynote symptoms of this remedy are:

✓ Thick yellow or green discharges
✓ Needs consolation
✓ Changeable temperament or symptoms
✓ A great remedy for ear infections or ear pain

◈ ◈ ◈ ◈ ◈

Other symptoms of Pulsatilla are:

Cause: Indulging in fatty or rich foods; becoming suddenly chilled when hot; getting wet

Mind: Sweet natured but can be self-pitying or irritable when sick; company makes patient better; needs comfort, better from crying and sympathy; emotional; shy; sensitive and easily hurt; moody and weeps easily; mild disposition; child weepy, whiny, clingy; indecisive; may fear death or germs

Head: Pain in temples; headache from indigestion; headache with burning tears on affected side; headache from overwork; vertigo when lying down, stooping; sitting, walking outdoors, and from using the eyes

Face: Flushed; right sided facial pain; face pain better from heat; lightness of forehead

Eyes: Thick, profuse, yellow-green discharge from eyes; inflamed lids; burning eyes; misty sight

Ears: Earache with pain shooting to teeth or lower jaw; plugged up; loss of hearing from fluid in ear; redness of external ear; throbbing pain; pus, blood, or yellow discharge from ears; deafness after measles

Nose: Inflamed mucus membranes; stuffed at night and indoors, flows in the open air; profuse discharge of mucus; running or blocked nose; sinus congestion; bland nasal discharge; stuffed up at night and copious flow in the morning; discharge may alternate from side to side; discharge fluent in open air but stuffed up in the house (opposite of Nux Vomica); or clear outside, stuffed up or flows outside; bloody discharge; loss of sense of smell; thick yellow or green discharge; nasal discharge worse at night

Mouth and Tongue: Chapped, peeling lips; dry mouth; may not be thirsty; licks lips often; bad bitter or salty taste in mouth; lips chap and peel; blisters on tongue; lower lip cracked in the middle; tongue coated yellow or white; loss of taste

Throat: Bluish red; stinging pain, worse swallowing; swollen throat; hard to swallow empty because throat feels constricted; red sore throat worse evening or afternoon

Larynx: Hoarseness that comes and goes

Neck and Back: Shooting pains nape and back; cracking in neck and upper back when moving

Chest: Feeling of pressure on chest; short of breath

Cough: Dry cough at night; worse lying down or at night; or patient coughs all day but ceases at night; dry, or productive yellow, green, thick, bitter or bland discharge; loose cough with greenish yellow phlegm; cough caused by breathing in; cough dry in the evening but loose in the morning; coughs from clearing the throat; cough worse lying down and forces him to sit up; coughing and gagging with thick yellow mucus

Extremities: Shooting pains in limbs, especially calves; chills in extremities; leg pain when hanging down; feels as if tendons are too short

Stomach: Distended, rumbling stomach; belching; stomach pains after eating

Food: Appetite changeable, either ravenous or absent; desires butter, ice cream, creamy food, peanut butter; aversion to fat, milk, and pork; aggravation from rich food; patient not thirsty, or has thirst before chills

Sleep: Sits up in bed because of cough; tendency to sleep during the day; talking in sleep; wakes frightened; sleeps with arms raised over head or crossed over abdomen

Fever: Chilliness; chills at 4:00 in the afternoon; chills of one side only, or only one side feels hot

Worse: Heat; humidity; warm room; warmth and overheated; too many coverings; evening and night; eating rich food; after eating; in the evening

Better: Outdoors; slow walking in open air; cool air; gentle motion

Generals: One sided complaints; chills begin in hands and feet and with pain in limbs; profuse sweats in the morning; one sided chilliness turns to one sided heat and turns into one sided sweat; patient wants fresh or cool air even when chilled; pains appear fast and go slowly, or appear slowly and leave quickly

Rhus Toxicodendron
(russ tocks-i-ko-den-drahn)

Rhus Toxicodendron is not one of the more common cold and flu remedies, but it is indicated a fair amount of the time for flu when body aches are better with motion or restlessness, especially at night.

Rhus Tox is better lying on something hard, similar to Bryonia, except that Rhus is better with motion and Bryonia is not.

The Rhus Toxicodendron plant is commonly known as poison ivy, and is used to treat that condition as well. It's also a good injury remedy for a painful back when rising in the morning but better with continued motion; however, if the motion goes on for a time the patient will then become stiff and sore again.

People who need Rhus Tox have a thick yellow discharge and tend to be very thirsty. You won't use Rhus Tox often for colds, but it should be considered when the symptoms agree and the bodily aches are better from movement.

◆ ◆ ◆ ◆ ◆

Keynote symptoms of Rhus Toxicodendron are:

✓ Body aches better from motion
✓ Thick yellow discharge from nose
✓ Thirsty

◆ ◆ ◆ ◆ ◆

Other symptoms of Rhus Tox include:

Cause: Overexertion; after getting wet; cold and damp weather; wet head; low activity (physical); getting wet while perspiring

Mind: Restless, especially at night; anxiety; sad at twilight; worried; patient forgets what he has started to do; desires solitude; low self-confidence; slow comprehension; cloudy sensation

Head: Dizziness worse when standing up or walking; vertigo and staggering to the right; vertigo worse in the morning; heavy head; headache worse on the right side; headache makes dull; migraine headaches better from taking a long walk outdoors; head pain worse from coughing

Face: Pale; jaws crack when chewing; face pain worse in the evening; swollen face

Eyes: Swollen eyes and lids; red eyes; eyes sore when moving; profuse, stinging tears; lids stuck together in the morning; sties

Ears: Pain in ears; sensation as if something is in them; feels as if wind is blowing in the ear (similar to Nux Vomica)

Nose: Yellow, thick discharge; violent discharge; dry stuffiness; sneezing; tip of nose red, sore, and ulcerated; swollen nose; nosebleed with dark blood

Mouth and Tongue: Red, triangular tip of tongue; tongue dry, red, brownish; yawning; dry tongue; tongue coated white; jaws crackle while chewing; lips and mouth dry; lips cracked

Throat: Feels swollen or bruised; mucus in throat; hawking of mucus; sticking pain on swallowing; dry throat

Larynx: Cold may go into larynx; hoarseness, burning pain in larynx; better using the voice

Neck and Back: Swollen glands; swollen parotid glands; stiff neck; stiff or painful lower back

Chest: Chest pain when coughing

Cough: Cough dry; patient coughs in sleep; cough from least movement; cough with vomiting; hard cough; expectoration of bright red blood; cough worse midnight to morning; coughs when putting hands out of bed

Extremities: Muscle aches and stiffness; stiffness so severe he feels paralyzed; colds settle in body and limbs; achy bones; muscle weakness; calf cramps; tearing pains in ligaments and tendons; stiffness and lameness

Stomach: Pressure and fullness, distention and bloating of abdomen; nausea, vertigo, and bloated abdomen after eating; gas

Food: Patient has no appetite but thirsty for cold drinks; craves cold milk, water, and oysters

Sleep: Tosses and turns in bed; heavy sleep; dreams of exertion

Fever: Evening fever; transient heat; patient perspires with heat; night sweats; chill followed by heat

Worse: Sitting in one position for a long time; cold cloth or applications; cold; cold fresh air; cold wet air after rain; during rest; undressing; lying right side; 7:00 in the evening

Better: Continuing to move; heat; hot sun; warm applications; massage; motion; lying on a hard floor; after change of position

Generals: Aches getting out of seat or out of bed; tearing pain; sensitive to cold drafts; skin itches; sensitive to cold air; sweats from taking warm drink

Sulphur
(sul-fur)

Although some older homeopaths disagree, Sulphur is one of the most common constitutional deep-acting remedies for chronic illness. So common is its use that if any hundred people are given Sulphur, a majority of them will improve because the remedy is so common.

Sulphur cases in general have an affinity for abstract thought—and sometimes mechanical aptitude. I remember a child patient I had who was a Sulphur case. The deciding factor was that at the age of five, she got her father's wrench and took the training wheels off her friend's bicycle so that she could have a two-wheeler!

I think it is more common to give Sulphur for a cold to those who seem to have a lot of Sulphur in their constitutions, who have the predisposition for abstract thought or mechanical aptitude. But, if you have neither of these characteristics and Sulphur fits the rest of your cold, don't be afraid to use it.

The old homeopaths used to say that Sulphur was untidy; nowadays, with our standards of hygiene, the untidiness is apt to be in one area of the patient's life: dresser drawers, back seat of the car, medicine chest, or other hidden area.

In terms of treating colds and flu, however, Sulphur is useful for particular kinds of colds and flu when the symptoms agree. It is like Belladonna in that it is dry, but Sulphur colds are not as violent in their onset as are Belladonna colds.

Periodicity is common in Sulphur ailments, with ailments re-occurring on a regular basis. Look for recurrent symptoms every seven to fourteen days, at the same time each day, or any other regular pattern.

Sometimes, Sulphur is also used to combat deep-rooted toxins, such as the bad effects of vaccination, pesticides, or drug use.

There are three textbook symptoms that may point you toward Sulphur. First, the person may feel that his feet are too hot under the covers and stick his feet out of bed at night. Secondly, he may be prone to early morning diarrhea that forces him out of bed. Third, he is very uncomfortable standing still, whether it be standing in line or standing to have clothes fitted. If your patient has these symptoms, look very carefully at Sulphur before you give another remedy.

If uncertain about a cold or flu and Anas Barbarae and Influenzinum don't fit, give Sulphur and wait to re-evaluate; often the symptoms will change to give you a clearer picture. Or, if your chosen remedy does not work, try Sulphur.

❖ ❖ ❖ ❖ ❖

The symptoms to watch for Sulphur are:

✓ Patient has affinity for abstract thought or mechanical aptitude
✓ Untidy in one area of his life
✓ Periodicity of symptoms
✓ Heat of bed covers makes patient put his feet out at night
✓ Early morning diarrhea that forces him out of bed

❖ ❖ ❖ ❖ ❖

Other symptoms of Sulphur include:

Cause: Overwork; partly recovers and then relapses; alcohol; getting chilled

Mind: Argumentative and speculative; not too tidy; dwells on religious, philosophical or abstract ideas; can be either selfish or extremely generous; lack of persistence; worries about future; poor memory

Head: Throbbing headache; heat on top of head with cold feet; feet burn at night in bed; headache better in warm room (contrary to rest of symptoms); head pain when coughing; headache from hunger; dizzy after meal, or exercising in the open air; stooping or looking down, going up ascent or rising from seat; pressure in head, especially on forehead; headache is worse out of doors; rebound headache after the week's work, on the weekend; sensation of a tight band around forehead; feels as if head is going to burst

Face: Burning face; red face without much fever; face pale or yellowish; face pain right half of face

Eyes: Heaviness and itching of lids; eye pain worse using eyes and in sunlight; profuse tears or eyes are dry; mucus in eyes; halo around lights; eyes burn; specks in front of eyes

Ears: Itching ears; pus and fluid in ears; humming in ears

Nose: Constant sneezing; thick yellow mucus; bloody nose when blown; nose bleeds in the morning with vertigo; stoppage of nose; acrid and burning nasal discharge; oversensitive to odors; dry stuffiness; scabs in nose; sense of smell either acute or lost; nose burns and itches; tip of nose red and shiny

Mouth and Tongue: Lips rough and dry; cracked; dry heat of mouth; red lips; tongue white with red tip and borders; mouth ulcers

Throat: Burning and dryness; chronic sore throat; tonsils enlarged or purple; rough, raw throat; pressure like plug in throat; difficulty swallowing as if ball in throat; sensation of hair or splinter in throat; burning, red, dry throat

Larynx: Sensation as if larynx is swollen or has a ball in it

Neck and Back: Stiff neck; pain in small of back; pain when rising from a chair; glands of neck swollen

Chest: Burning in or pressure on chest; short of breath; patient feels like he's suffocating when lying down; feels like he can't take in a full breath; pain obstructing left side of chest

Cough: Violent racking cough; bronchitis; night cough, cough with congested head; wet cough; watery yellow-green expectoration or milk white mucus; cough when breathing deep or talking

Extremities: Joint pain is better in the morning and worse in bed at night; tendency of limbs to go to sleep; legs heavy; stiff and painful joints, especially knees; cramps in soles and calves at night

Stomach: Burning pain in stomach; belching with bad taste in mouth; after a meal pressure in chest or stomach, nausea; cramps in stomach; distended stomach; gas; vomiting; heartburn and increased saliva

Food: Aversion to water, alcohol, eggs, squash, meat, rye bread, fat or milk; loss of appetite or excessive appetite; ravenous hunger with attacks of vomiting; weak and faint around 11:00 in the morning, needs something to eat; not hungry for breakfast; sits down to a meal and loses appetite; craves fat, spicy food, sweets, salt, pickles; also acids and sweets, or also has an aversion to these things; milk and eggs aggravate; milk leads to vomiting; patient does not eat in the morning but snacks during the day; very thirsty, especially for beer

Sleep: Drowsy in afternoon and evening; can't fall asleep or frequent waking; waking too early in the morning and sleeps in too long; talks, jerks, twitches in sleep; vivid dreams; can't sleep between 2:00 and 5:00 in the morning; sings in sleep; happy dreams

Fever: Red skin; chills with shivering; night sweats on nape of neck and back of head

Worse: In the morning; from alcohol, damp and cold or very hot weather; washing; warmth of bed; prolonged sitting or standing; 11:00 in the morning; in the spring (they get colds); study, in the night, 12:00 midnight or noon; severe cold; oversleeping

Better: Dry, warm weather; lying on the right side; fresh air, dry air; likes the feel of cold air; sitting and lying

Generals: Stool loose and burning; rectal itching; diarrhea with gas; ear canals, anus, nostrils, may be bright red; disturbed heat; warm hands, cold feet, or vice versa; sensitive to open air; sweats profusely, sweat smells sour; anus sore; constipation alternating with diarrhea; talking fatigues and makes headache worse; head and stomach worse in the open air; frequent and profuse perspiring; skin itches; perspiration may smell sour

Part Four:

A Cold And Flu Repertory

Back:

Chills Down Back:
    Allium Cepa
Cracking:
    Upper Back, When Moving:
        Pulsatilla Nigricans
Stiffness:
    Anas Barbarae
    Ferrum Phosphoricum
    Phosphorus
Pain:
    Bryonia
    Eupatorium Perfoliatum
    Natrum Muriaticum
    Better Heat:
        Bryonia
    Better Firm Support:
        Bryonia
        Natrum Muriaticum
    When:
        3:00-4:00 In The Morning:
            Pulsatilla Nigricans
        When Rising From A Chair:
            Sulphur
    Where:
        Coccyx:
            Phosphorus
        Hip Joints:
            Aconitum Napellus
        Lower Back:
            Rhus Toxicodendron
        Pelvis:
            Aconitum Napellus
        Shoulder:
            Ferrum Phosphoricum
        Shoulder Blades:
            Shooting Pain
                Hepar Sulphuris
                Calcareum

Small Of Back:
        Calcarea Carbonica
        Sulphur
Tail Bone:
        Kali Bichromicum
Quality:
        Aching Pain:
                Eupatorium Perfoliatum*
        Bruised Pain:
                Aconitum Napellus
        Burning Pain:
                Phosphorus
        Dull Ache:
                Gelsemium Sempervirens
        Shooting Pain:
                Pulsatilla Nigricans
Worse:
        Sitting:
                Kali Bichromicum
        Walking:
                Kali Bichromicum

Better:

Bathing:
> Washing Face:
> > Ferrum Phosphoricum

Clothing:
> Bundling Up:
> > Hepar Sulphuris Calcareum
> Loose Clothes:
> > Lycopodium Clavatum

Company:
> Being With Other People:
> > Phosphorus
> Left Alone:
> > Nux Vomica

Environment:
> Asthma Better Outdoors, All Else Worse:
> > Nux Vomica
> Cold Room:
> > Bryonia
> Cool Air:
> > Lycopodium Clavatum
> > Pulsatilla Nigricans
> Cool Surroundings:
> > Allium Cepa
> Dry Air:
> > Sulphur
> Dry, Warm Weather:
> > Sulphur
> Fresh Air:
> > Allium Cepa
> > Sulphur
> Hot Sun:
> > Rhus Toxicodendron
> In Cold Rain:
> > Allium Cepa*
> Fresh Air:
> > Aconitum Napellus*
> Moist, Wet Weather (Opposite Of Gelsemium Sempervirens):

Hepar Sulphuris Calcareum

Open Air:
Aconitum Napellus
Bryonia
Gelsemium Sempervirens
Natrum Muriaticum
Phosphorus
Open Air (Even Though They Caught The Cold From A Draft):
Natrum Muriaticum
Outdoors:
Allium Cepa*
Pulsatilla Nigricans
Outdoors (Even Though Nose Stopped Up):
Arsenicum Album
The Feel Of Cold Air:
Sulphur
Warm Room:
Hepar Sulphuris Calcareum
Wet Weather:
Nux Vomica

Fluid:
Expectorating Fluid:
Kali Bichromicum

Food And Drink:
After Eating Vegetables:
Arsenicum Album
Alcohol:
Gelsemium Sempervirens
Cold Food And Drink:
Bryonia
Eating:
Gelsemium Sempervirens
Lycopodium Clavatum
Hot Drinks:
Hepar Sulphuris Calcareum
Stimulants:
Gelsemium Sempervirens
Warm Drinks:

Arsenicum Album
Lycopodium Clavatum
Warm Food And Drink:
Arsenicum Album

Motion:

Continued Motion:
Gelsemium Sempervirens
Rhus Toxicodendron*
Gentle Exercise:
Ferrum Phosphoricum
Gentle Motion:
Ferrum Phosphoricum
Pulsatilla Nigricans
Massage:
Phosphorus
Rhus Toxicodendron
Movement:
Kali Bichromicum
Lycopodium Clavatum
Not Moving In A Warm Room:
Belladonna
Slow Walking In The Open Air:
Pulsatilla Nigricans

Perspiring:

Gelsemium Sempervirens

Position:

After Change In Position:
Rhus Toxicodendron
Bending Forward:
Gelsemium Sempervirens
Bending The Head Backwards:
Belladonna
Getting Out Of Bed:
Vertigo And Headache Better, But Cough Is
Worse When He Gets Out Of Bed:
Natrum Muriaticum
Kneeling With Face Towards Pillow:
Eupatorium Perfoliatum
Lying Down:
Nux Vomica

Kali Bichromicum
Sulphur
Lying Down In A Dark Place:
    Belladonna
Lying Down: Makes Vertigo And Headache
Better But Cough Worse:
    Natrum Muriaticum
Lying On Hard Floor:
    Rhus Toxicodendron
Lying On Right Side:
    Phosphorus
    Sulphur
Lying Still:
    Gelsemium Sempervirens
    Lying Still And Being Left Alone:
    Bryonia*
On Hands And Knees:
    Eupatorium Perfoliatum
Sitting:
    Phosphorus
    Sulphur
    Sitting Upright In A Dark Room:
    Belladonna
Standing In A Dark Room:
    Belladonna

Pressure:
Firm Pressure:
    Nux Vomica
Physical Pressure:
    Gelsemium Sempervirens

Sleep:
Sleep, After:
    Aconitum Napellus
    After Adequate Unbroken Sleep:
        Nux Vomica
    Sound Sleep:
        Phosphorus

Rest:
Anas Barbarae
Mercurius Vivus

Temperature:
Cold Cloth Or Ice Pack:
    Ferrum Phosphoricum
Getting Cold:
    Lycopodium Clavatum
Heat:
    Anas Barbarae
    Arsenicum Album
    Hepar Sulphuris Calcareum
    Kali Bichromicum
    Rhus Toxicodendron
Warmth:
    Belladonna
    Nux Vomica
    Warm Applications/Compresses:
        Phosphorus
        Rhus Toxicodendron
        Belladonna
        Hepar Sulphuris Calcareum

Time:
In The Evening:
    Nux Vomica
Morning:
    Mercurius Vivus

Urinating:
After Profuse Urination:
    Gelsemium Sempervirens*

Causes And Onset: (See also Generalities: Cold Traits)

Alcohol:
 Calcarea Carbonica
 Sulphur

Chill:
 Aconitum Napellus*
 Sulphur
 Pulsatilla Nigricans
 Chill After Sweating:
  Aconitum Napellus*
  Calcarea
 Chill To The Head, Haircut
  Belladonna
  Phosphorus
 Chill In Water:
  Arsenicum Album
  Calcarea Carbonica

Divorce:
 Natrum Muriaticum

Drugs:
 Nux Vomica*

Environment:
 Change Of Weather:
  Gelsemium Sempervirens
 Cold To Warm:
  Bryonia
 Cold Weather Or Air:
  Allium Cepa
  Belladonna
 Cold, Damp Weather:
  Allium Cepa
  Rhus Toxicodendron
 Cold, Dry Wind Or Weather:
  Aconitum Napellus*
  Gelsemium Sempervirens
  Hepar Sulphuris Calcareum
  Nux Vomica

Drafts:
    Natrum Muriaticum
Getting Wet:
    Pulsatilla Nigricans
Getting Wet While Perspiring:
    Rhus Toxicodendron
Heat Of The Sun:
    Aconitum Napellus
Warm Wet Weather:
    Gelsemium Sempervirens
Wind:
    After Perspiration:
        Aconitum Napellus*
Wet Wind:
    Belladonna

Exhaustion
    Calcarea Carbonica
    Nux Vomica*
Food Poisoning:
    Arsenicum Album
Haircut, Chill To The Head:
    Belladonna
    Phosphorus
Hay Fever:
    Allium Cepa*
    Euphrasia Officinalis
Immune System
Immune System Weak, Prone To Chronic Colds:
    Arsenicum Album*
    Calcarea*
    Sulphur*
Injury:
    Aconitum Napellus
Lack Of Sleep:
    Nux Vomica
Medicine:
    Nux Vomica
Mental:
    Anger:
        Bryonia

       Lycopodium Clavatum
       Natrum Muriaticum*
       Nux Vomica*

Anxiety:
       Lycopodium Clavatum

Embarrassment:
       Bryonia
       Gelsemium Sempervirens
       Lycopodium Clavatum

Fright:
       Aconitum Napellus*
       Arsenicum Album
       Bryonia
       Calcarea Carbonica
       Gelsemium Sempervirens
       Lycopodium Clavatum
       Natrum Muriaticum
       Mercurius Vivus

Grief:
       Arsenicum Album
       Natrum Muriaticum*

Rejection:
       Natrum Muriaticum

Resentment:
       Bryonia

Shock:
       Aconitum Napellus
       Gelsemium Sempervirens
       Natrum Muriaticum*

Stress:
       Natrum Muriaticum
       Nux Vomica*

Unrequited Love:
       Natrum Muriaticum

Onset:
Exposure To Cold With Onset The Same Day:
       Aconitum Napellus*
First Pick For Onset Of Influenza:
       Anas Barbarae*
       Influenzinum*

Hot, Dry, Sudden, Violent:
> Belladonna*

Sudden:
> Aconitum Napellus*

When You Are Too Rushed To Find The Specific
Remedy For Flu:
> Anas Barbarae*
> Influenzinum*

Overexertion, Overwork:
Ferrum Phosphoricum
Nux Vomica*
Rhus Toxicodendron
Sulphur

Overindulgence:
Beer:
> Kali Bichromicum

Coffee:
> Nux Vomica*

Fatty Or Rich Foods:
> Pulsatilla Nigricans

Food Or Drink:
> Nux Vomica

Malt Beverages:
> Kali Bichromicum

Wine:
> Lycopodium Clavatum

Relapses After Partial Recovery:
Sulphur

Seasonal Allergies:
Allium Cepa*

Seasons:
Spring And Autumn:
> Kali Bichromicum

Spring Colds:
> Allium Cepa

Summer Colds:
> Gelsemium Sempervirens

Winters:
> Mild:
>> Gelsemium Sempervirens

Sedentary, Low Activity:
Nux Vomica
Rhus Toxicodendron
Stimulants:
Nux Vomica
Stomach Flu:
Arsenicum Album
Surgery:
Aconitum Napellus
Swimming In Sea Water:
Arsenicum Album
Taking On Too Much Responsibility:
Arsenicum Album
Bryonia
Calcarea Carbonica
Gelsemium Sempervirens
Lycopodium Clavatum
Natrum Muriaticum
Mercurius Vivus
Tobacco Smoke:
Arsenicum Album

Chest:

Breath:
Difficult, Hard To Breathe:
Aconitum Napellus
Bryonia
Mercurius Vivus
Hot:
Aconitum Napellus
Noisy Respiration:
Phosphorus
Oppressed:
Ferrum Phosphoricum
Panting:
Ferrum Phosphoricum
Phosphorus
Shallow:
Nux Vomica
Short Of Breath:
Aconitum Napellus
Arsenicum Album
Belladonna
Euphrasia Officinalis
Ferrum Phosphoricum
Hepar Sulphuris Calcareum
Mercurius Vivus
Nux Vomica
Pulsatilla Nigricans
Sulphur
When Going Upstairs:
Calcarea Carbonica
Slightest Effort Makes Them Short Of Breath:
Calcarea Carbonica
Shortness Of Breath Worse Night And Morning:
Nux Vomica
Slow:
Gelsemium Sempervirens
Snoring Breathing:

Belladonna
Wheezing:
Arsenicum Album
Lycopodium Clavatum
Burning:
Arsenicum Album
Lycopodium Clavatum
Sulphur
Colds Go To Chest With Lots Of Phlegm:
Allium Cepa
Constrictive:
Arsenicum Album
Nux Vomica
Diseases:
Bronchitis:
Lycopodium Clavatum
Mercurius Vivus
Acute Bronchitis:
Gelsemium Sempervirens
Pleurisy:
Phosphorus
Esp. Of Right Lung:
Phosphorus
Pneumonia After Flu:
Gelsemium Sempervirens
Unresolved Pneumonia:
Lycopodium Clavatum
Empty Feeling In Chest:
Phosphorus
Feels Like He Can't Take A Full Breath:
Sulphur
Feels Like Suffocating When Lying Down:
Sulphur
Heaviness:
Lycopodium Clavatum
Pain:
Ferrum Phosphoricum
Natrum Muriaticum
Phosphorus
Sore Pain:

Gelsemium Sempervirens
Hepar Sulphuris Calcareum
Darting Pain Upper Third Of Right Lung:
Arsenicum Album
Left Side Of Chest:
Phosphorus
Sulphur
Stabbing Pain Right Lung To Back:
Mercurius Vivus
Throbbing Pain:
Lycopodium Clavatum
Wet Weather:
After Exposure To Wet Weather:
Calcarea Carbonica
When Coughing:
Rhus Toxicodendron
With Dry Hacking Cough:
Ferrum Phosphoricum
Stitching Pain When Breathing In:
Aconitum Napellus
Bryonia
Eupatorium Perfoliatum
Phlegm/Fluid:
Fluid Hard To Cough Up:
Bryonia
Tenacious Fluid:
Hepar Sulphuris Calcareum
Rattling Of Phlegm In Chest:
Hepar Sulphuris Calcareum
Especially In Sleep:
Hepar Sulphuris Calcareum
Pressure:
Bryonia
Sulphur
Pulsatilla Nigricans
Pressure Better After Rising:
Kali Bichromicum
Sensitive To Pressure:
Calcarea Carbonica
Tight:

Aconitum Napellus
Phosphorus
Weight On Chest:
Phosphorus

Cough:

Better:

At Night:
Ferrum Phosphoricum
Bending The Head Backwards:
Hepar Sulphuris Calcareum
Cold Drinks:
Phosphorus
Lying Down, But Nasal Discharge Worse:
Euphrasia Officinalis

Cause:

Breathing In:
Pulsatilla Nigricans
Clearing The Throat:
Pulsatilla Nigricans
Cold Wind:
Aconitum Napellus
Coughs When Body Part Is Uncovered:
Hepar Sulphuris Calcareum
Coughs From Least Movement:
Rhus Toxicodendron
Pain In Larynx:
Hepar Sulphuris Calcareum
Putting Hands Out Of Bed:
Rhus Toxicodendron

Cough, General:

Anas Barbarae

Cough (Type Of Cough And Time)

At Night:
Sulphur
Barking Cough With Sore Chest:
Eupatorium Perfoliatum
Barking:
Belladonna
Hepar Sulphuris Calcareum
Brassy Cough:
Kali Bichromicum
Coughs All Day But Ceases At Night:
Pulsatilla Nigricans

Dry Cough:
>Belladonna
>Bryonia*
>Ferrum Phosphoricum
>Gelsemium Sempervirens
>Mercurius Vivus
>Phosphorus*
>Pulsatilla Nigricans
>Rhus Toxicodendron
>Dry And Loose:
>>Hepar Sulphuris Calcareum
>>At Night:
>>>Pulsatilla Nigricans
>>Constant:
>>>Aconitum Napellus
>Hacking Cough:
>>Arsenicum Album
>>Ferrum Phosphoricum
>>Nux Vomica
>Dry In The Evening But Loose In The Morning:
>>Pulsatilla Nigricans
>Dry, Tearing:
>>Nux Vomica
>Dry, Tearing Cough That Scrapes Throat:
>>Belladonna
>First Dry, Then Loose:
>>Phosphorus

Exhausting:
>Phosphorus

Gagging:
>Hepar Sulphuris Calcareum
>Pulsatilla Nigricans

Hard:
>Rhus Toxicodendron

Loose:
>Pulsatilla Nigricans
>Loose, Rattling, Sensation Of Strangling:

Hepar Sulphuris Calcareum

Loud Cough:
  Aconitum Napellus

Makes Chest Hurt:
  Bryonia

No Cough:
  No Cough At Night:
    Euphrasia Officinalis

Persistent:
  Phosphorus

Raspy:
  Phosphorus

Rough:
  Mercurius Vivus

Short:
  Short Cough:
    Belladonna
  Short Chronic Cough:
    Natrum Muriaticum
  Short Dry Cough With Tickling In Throat:
    Aconitum Napellus
  Short, Painful:
    Ferrum Phosphoricum

Sporadic With Soreness Of Chest:
  Nux Vomica

Sudden Cough:
  Belladonna

Teasing And Tickling:
  Gelsemium Sempervirens
  Tickling:
    Belladonna
    Mercurius Vivus
    Natrum Muriaticum
    Phosphorus

Violent Racking Cough:
  Sulphur

Wet Cough:
  Belladonna
  Euphrasia Officinalis

Sulphur
With Profuse Phlegm:
> Euphrasia Officinalis

With Tenacious Mucus:
> Bryonia

Wheezing:
> Arsenicum Album

Whistling Cough:
> Aconitum Napellus

Whooping:
> Belladonna

Expectoration:
Lycopodium Clavatum
Bloody:
> Arsenicum Album
> Mercurius Vivus
> Bright Red Blood:
>> Arsenicum Album
>> Rhus Toxicodendron
>
> Sputum Blood Streaked:
>> Aconitum Napellus
>
> Frothy:
>> Arsenicum Album

Green:
> Pulsatilla Nigricans
> Green And Thick:
>> Mercurius Vivus

Greenish-Yellow:
> Pulsatilla Nigricans

Rusty Discharge:
> Phosphorus

Spits Nothing Up:
> Aconitum Napellus

Thick:
> Mercurius Vivus

Watery Yellow-Green Expectoration:
> Sulphur

Wet Cough Daytime With Expectoration, Dry
Cough At Night With No Expectoration:
> Lycopodium Clavatum

Mucus/Phlegm:
  Bitter:
      Pulsatilla Nigricans
  Bland:
      Pulsatilla Nigricans
  Bloody Mucus:
      Natrum Muriaticum
  Can't Bring Anything Up:
      Bryonia*
      Hepar Sulphuris Calcareum
  Color:
          Greenish-Yellow:
              Pulsatilla Nigricans
          Milk White Mucus:
              Sulphur
          Yellow Phlegm:
              Phosphorus
              Pulsatilla Nigricans
              Thick Yellow:
                  Hepar Sulphuris
                  Calcareum
                  Thick, Yellow, Sweet
                  Tasting:
                      Calcarea Carbonica
  Lots Of Mucus:
      Belladonna
      Euphrasia Officinalis
  Tastes Salty Or Sweet:
      Phosphorus
  Tenacious Mucus Hard To Dislodge:
      Bryonia
  Thick:
      Anas Barbarae
      Pulsatilla Nigricans
Onset:
  Not Useful In The Beginning Stages Of Cough:
      Kali Bichromicum
PostureAnd Position:
  Position:

Coughs With One Hand On Chest, The
Other On Head:
>Bryonia*

Presses Hand To The Sternum While
Coughing:
>Bryonia

When:

Asleep:
>Rhus Toxicodendron

Breathing Deep:
>Sulphur

Talking:
>Sulphur

Waking Up:
>Wakes Up With Croupy Cough:
>>Aconitum Napellus
>
>Wakes Up With Dry Cough:
>>Aconitum Napellus
>
>Wakes Up With Loose Cough:
>>Aconitum Napellus

With (Cough With):

Choking:
>Mercurius Vivus

Congested Head:
>Sulphur

Retching Or Vomiting:
>Retching:
>>Mercurius Vivus
>>Nux Vomica
>>Phosphorus
>>Ends In Retching:
>>>Nux Vomica
>
>Vomiting:
>>Mercurius Vivus
>>Phosphorus
>>Rhus Toxicodendron
>
>Retching And Vomiting:
>>Ferrum Phosphoricum
>>Natrum Muriaticum

Worse:

After Taking A Deep Breath:
    Bryonia
Drinking:
    Aconitum Napellus
    Arsenicum Album
    Bryonia
    Drinking Anything Cold:
        Hepar Sulphuris Calcareum
Eating:
    Aconitum Napellus
    Anything Cold:
    Hepar Sulphuris Calcareum
    After Eating:
        Bryonia
Environment:
    Being Out Of Doors:
        Arsenicum Album
    Cold Air:
        Ferrum Phosphoricum
        Hepar Sulphuris Calcareum
        Phosphorus
    Open Air:
        Phosphorus
Going Upstairs:
    Calcarea Carbonica
Hard And Dry Cough Worse At Night:
    Bryonia
Laughing:
    Bryonia
    Phosphorus
Strong Odors:
    Phosphorus
Mental:
    Emotional Upset:
        Aconitum Napellus
Position:
    Lying Down:
        Aconitum Napellus
        Lying Down, And Forces Him To
        Sit Up:

Pulsatilla Nigricans
Lying Down:
 Cough Worse Lying Down:
Calcarea Carbonica
Lying On Left Side:
Phosphorus
Talking:
Belladonna
Bryonia
Phosphorus
Tobacco Smoke:
Aconitum Napellus
Bryonia
Time:
Daytime:
Euphrasia Officinalis
Evening:
4:00-6:00 In The Evening:
Lycopodium Clavatum
Evening Until Midnight:
Hepar Sulphuris Calcareum
Midnight To Morning:
Rhus Toxicodendron
Morning:
Kali Bichromicum
2:00 And 4:00 In The Morning:
Eupatorium Perfoliatum
Night:
Belladonna
Mercurius Vivus
Night With Wheezing
Tickling Cough Worse Night:
Calcarea Carbonica
Respiration:
Arsenicum Album

Ears: (Inner Ear)

Boils Inside Ear Canal:
> Hepar Sulphuris Calcareum

Congestion:
> Lycopodium Clavatum
> Sulphur
> Blockage Of Eustachian Tube From Mucus:
>> Nux Vomica
> Fluid In Middle Ear:
>> Calcarea Carbonica
>> Swallows Frequently For Relief:
>>> Nux Vomica
> Plugged Up:
>> Pulsatilla Nigricans

Discharges:
> Bloody:
>> Hepar Sulphuris Calcareum
>> Pulsatilla Nigricans
> Burning:
>> Mercurius Vivus
> Mucus:
>> Yellow:
>>> Phosphorus
>>> Pulsatilla Nigricans
>> Thick, Yellow, Offensive Discharge:
>>> Lycopodium Clavatum
>> Thin, Burning, Offensive Smelling:
>>> Arsenicum Album
>>> Nux Vomica
> Pus:
>> Allium Cepa
>> Belladonna
>> Hepar Sulphuris Calcareum*
>> Mercurius Vivus
>> Pulsatilla Nigricans
>> Sulphur

Infection:
> Hepar Sulphuris Calcareum
> Pulsatilla Nigricans*

Infections Of Children:
>> Belladonna*

Itching:
Hepar Sulphuris Calcareum
Nux Vomica
Sulphur

Hearing:
Deafness:
>> After Measles:
>>>> Pulsatilla Nigricans
>> From Ear Fluid:
>>>> Pulsatilla Nigricans
>> With Cold:
>>>> Phosphorus
>> Difficulty Hearing Human Voice:
>>>> Phosphorus
>> Dull Hearing:
>>>> Belladonna
>> Hypersensitive To Noise:
>>>> Aconitum Napellus
>>>> To Children Playing:
>>>>>> Arsenicum Album
>> Sounds Reverberate:
>>>> Belladonna
>> Super Acute Hearing:
>>>> Belladonna
>>>> Loud Sounds Painful:
>>>>>> Nux Vomica
>>>> Music Unbearable:
>>>>>> Aconitum Napellus
>> Tinnitus:
>>>> Aconitum Napellus
>>>> Lycopodium Clavatum

Pain:
Belladonna
Bryonia
Calcarea Carbonica
Kali Bichromicum
Pulsatilla Nigricans*
Rhus Toxicodendron

After Cold:
> Aconitum Napellus

Better From Warm Applications:
> Aconitum Napellus

Earaches:
> Allium Cepa
> Ferrum Phosphoricum
> Especially First Stage:
>> Ferrum Phosphoricum
> Especially In Children:
>> Belladonna

In Eardrums:
> Euphrasia Officinalis
> Nux Vomica

In The Cold:
> Gelsemium Sempervirens

Left Ear:
> Kali Bichromicum

Right Ear:
> Belladonna

Shooting Pain:
> Gelsemium Sempervirens
>> Eustachian Tubes:
> Allium Cepa
> Gelsemium Sempervirens

Extending Into Roof Of Mouth:
> Kali Bichromicum

Shoots Into Lower Jaw:
> Pulsatilla Nigricans

Shoots Into Teeth:
> Pulsatilla Nigricans

Stinging Pain Shooting Into Head:
> Kali Bichromicum

Tearing Pain:
> Mercurius Vivus

Throbbing Pain:
> Pulsatilla Nigricans

When Blowing Nose:
> Hepar Sulphuris Calcareum

When Swallowing:

Gelsemium Sempervirens
Hepar Sulphuris Calcareum
Nux Vomica

Sounds In Ears:
Bells:
Arsenicum Album
Buzzing:
Aconitum Napellus
Bryonia
Ferrum Phosphoricum
Crackling In Ears:
Calcarea Carbonica
Nux Vomica
Hissing:
Nux Vomica
Humming:
Lycopodium Clavatum
Sulphur
Ringing:
Aconitum Napellus
Arsenicum Album
Ferrum Phosphoricum
Nux Vomica
Roaring:
Bryonia
Gelsemium Sempervirens
Lycopodium Clavatum
Mercurius Vivus
Natrum Muriaticum
Nux Vomica
Rushing:
Gelsemium Sempervirens
Stopped Up:
Bryonia
Ulcers In Ears:
Lycopodium Clavatum

Ears: (Outer Ears)

Hot:

Aconitum Napellus
Kali Bichromicum
Eczema Behind And Around Ear:
Lycopodium Clavatum
Itching:
Hepar Sulphuris Calcareum
Sulphur
Painful:
Aconitum Napellus
Red:
Aconitum Napellus
Pulsatilla Nigricans
Scabs:
Around Ear:
Hepar Sulphuris Calcareum
Behind Ear:
Hepar Sulphuris Calcareum
Swollen:
Aconitum Napellus

Extremities:

Chills In Extremities:
Pulsatilla Nigricans
Cracking:
Cracking In Joints:
Kali Bichromicum
Cramps:
Calves:
Calcarea Carbonica
Nux Vomica
Rhus Toxicodendron
Calves And Soles At Night:
Sulphur
Foot:
Calcarea Carbonica
Forearms:
Gelsemium Sempervirens
Legs:
Arsenicum Album
Limbs:
Phosphorus
Thighs:
Calcarea Carbonica
Hangnails:
Natrum Muriaticum
Hot And Cold:
Cold Extremities With Hot Head And Back:
Gelsemium Sempervirens
Cold Extremities With Rest Of Body Hot:
Ferrum Phosphoricum
Cold Feet:
Mercurius Vivus
Cold Feet Or One Hot And The Other Cold:
Lycopodium Clavatum
Cold Or Hot Hands:
Phosphorus
Hot Hands With Cold Feet:
Aconitum Napellus
Hot Head With Cold Extremities:

Belladonna
Hot Palms:
Natrum Muriaticum
Itchy Palms:
Hepar Sulphuris Calcareum
Jerking:
Jerking In Arms And Fingers:
Mercurius Vivus
Numbness:
Euphrasia Officinalis
Arms:
Aconitum Napellus
Legs:
Aconitum Napellus
Easily Numb:
Arms, Fingers, Hands:
Phosphorus
Pain:
Bones:
Eupatorium Perfoliatum*
Rhus Toxicodendron
Bruised:
Kali Bichromicum
Burning Pain:
Belladonna
Night:
Especially At Night In Bed:
Mercurius Vivus
Pain Changes Location In Limbs Quickly:
Kali Bichromicum
Stinging Pain:
Belladonna
Shooting Pains:
Belladonna
Tearing Pain:
Calcarea Carbonica
Location:
Arms And Hands:
Bryonia
Arms, Wrists, And Hands, Aching:

Eupatorium Perfoliatum
Bone Pain:
Calves:
Pulsatilla Nigricans
Calf, Foot, Thigh:
Pulsatilla Nigricans
Calf Tendons:
Kali Bichromicum
Hip And Knee:
Shooting Pain:
Aconitum Napellus
Joints:
Calcarea Carbonica
Lycopodium Clavatum
Mercurius Vivus
Sulphur
Joint Pain In Cold Damp Weather:
Calcarea Carbonica
Joint Pain Better In The Morning
And Worse In Bed At Night:
Sulphur
Joint Pain In Hip, Knees, Feet:
Calcarea Carbonica
Knees:
Sulphur
Legs:
Shooting Pain:
Euphrasia Officinalis
Ligaments And Tendons:
Rhus Toxicodendron
Limbs:
Bryonia
Shooting Pain In Limbs:
Pulsatilla Nigricans
Muscles:
Anas Barbarae
Gelsemium Sempervirens
Rhus Toxicodendron
Muscles Sore As If Beaten:
Eupatorium Perfoliatum

Muscles Sore As If Burning:
Ferrum Phosphoricum
Shoulders And Arms:
Rheumatic Pain:
Nux Vomica
Thighs:
Sticking Pain:
Euphrasia Officinalis
Wrists:
Nux Vomica
Wrists Hurt As If Broken:
Eupatorium Perfoliatum
Pain Worse:
Cold Weather:
Hepar Sulphuris Calcareum

Stiffness:
Rhus Toxicodendron
Phosphorus
Stiffness So Severe They Feel Paralyzed:
Rhus Toxicodendron
Location:
Elbows And Wrists:
Lycopodium Clavatum
Knees:
Lycopodium Clavatum

Sweating:
Cold Perspiration In Hands:
Hepar Sulphuris Calcareum
Icy Cold Palms:
Aconitum Napellus
Feet:
Mercurius Vivus
Palms:
Natrum Muriaticum
Mercurius Vivus

Swelling/Puffy:
Calcarea Carbonica
Joints:
Ferrum Phosphoricum

Painless Swelling Of Fingers And Hands:
Euphrasia Officinalis

Tingling:
Arms:
Aconitum Napellus
Legs:
Aconitum Napellus
Go To Sleep:
Arms And Legs:
Nux Vomica
Legs Go To Sleep When Sitting:
Calcarea Carbonica
Limbs:
Sulphur

Trembling:
Gelsemium Sempervirens
Mercurius Vivus

Weak/Weary:
Arms And Hands:
Bryonia
Legs Heavy:
Sulphur
Limbs Weak:
Gelsemium Sempervirens
Hepar Sulphuris Calcareum
Mercurius Vivus
Nux Vomica
Sulphur
Loss Of Power And Muscle Control:
Gelsemium Sempervirens
Muscle Weakness:
Rhus Toxicodendron

Eyes:

Burning:
>Calcarea Carbonica
>Sulphur
>Pulsatilla Nigricans

Conjunctivitis:
>Bryonia
>Euphrasia Officinalis
>Ferrum Phosphoricum
>Hepar Sulphuris Calcareum
>Conjunctivitis With Sticky Discharge:
>>Hepar Sulphuris Calcareum

Discharges:
>Acrid And Thick:
>>Euphrasia Officinalis
>Mucus:
>>Lycopodium Clavatum
>>Sulphur
>>Sticky Mucus In The Corners:
>>>Euphrasia Officinalis
>>Sticky Mucus On The Cornea:
>>>Euphrasia Officinalis
>>Yellow-Green Mucus:
>>>Pulsatilla Nigricans
>>Yellow Matter In The Corners Of Eyes:
>>>Kali Bichromicum

Dry:
>Aconitum Napellus
>Euphrasia Officinalis
>Lycopodium Clavatum
>Nux Vomica
>Sulphur

Hot:
>Aconitum Napellus

Itchy:
>Allium Cepa

Light:
>Needs Lots Of Light:
>>Aconitum Napellus

                    Gelsemium Sempervirens

Light Sensitive (Photophobia)
                    Aconitum Napellus
                    Allium Cepa
                    Arsenicum Album
                    Calcarea Carbonica
                    Euphrasia Officinalis
                    Eupatorium
                    Gelsemium Sempervirens
                    Hepar Sulphuris Calcareum
                    Kali Bichromicum
                    Mercurius Vivus
                    Especially In The Morning:
                         Nux Vomica

Pain:

Aching:
              Euphrasia Officinalis
              Lycopodium Clavatum

Bruised:
              Gelsemium Sempervirens
              Natrum Muriaticum

Painful Movement:
              Bryonia
              Hepar Sulphuris Calcareum
              Rhus Toxicodendron

Painful And Stiff Movement:
              Hepar Sulphuris Calcareum

Sore:
              Eupatorium Perfoliatum

Sore From Heat:
              Mercurius Vivus

Sore To The Touch:
              Phosphorus

Pupils:

Contracted:
              Nux Vomica

Dilated:
              Belladonna*
              Gelsemium Sempervirens
              Mercurius Vivus

Nux Vomica
One Dilated, The Other Constricted:
Gelsemium Sempervirens
Glassy:
Belladonna
Pressure:
Calcarea Carbonica
Euphrasia Officinalis
Hepar Sulphuris Calcareum
Rubs Eyes:
Allium Cepa
Red:
Aconitum Napellus
Allium Cepa
Arsenicum Album
Euphrasia Officinalis
Kali Bichromicum
Mercurius Vivus
Rhus Toxicodendron
Squinting:
Belladonna
Stinging:
Allium Cepa
Swollen:
Rhus Toxicodendron
Tearing:
Aconitum Napellus
Allium Cepa
Phosphorus
Acrid:
Mercurius Vivus
Burning/Stinging:
Arsenicum Album
Euphrasia Officinalis*
Mercurius Vivus
Rhus Toxicodendron
Cold And Windy Weather:
Euphrasia Officinalis
Profuse:
Euphrasia Officinalis

Kali Bichromicum
Mercurius Vivus
Natrum Muriaticum
Sulphur
Rhus Toxicodendron
Profuse, Bland:
Allium Cepa
Sunlight, In Sunlight:
Bryonia
When Coughing:
Natrum Muriaticum
When Laughing:
Natrum Muriaticum*

Vision:
Blurred:
Gelsemium Sempervirens
Distorted:
Belladonna
Disturbances In Vision:
Phosphorus
Double:
Gelsemium Sempervirens
Halo Around Lights:
Sulphur
Night Blindness:
Lycopodium Clavatum
Spots Or Specks:
Aconitum Napellus
Nux Vomica
Sulphur
Vision Better In Twilight:
Phosphorus

Eyelids:
Burning:
Kali Bichromicum
Droopy:
Gelsemium Sempervirens
Dry:

Nux Vomica
Heavy:
Gelsemium Sempervirens
Sulphur
Heavy In The Morning:
Kali Bichromicum
Hot:
Aconitum Napellus
Inflamed:
Pulsatilla Nigricans
Itchy:
Calcarea Carbonica
Kali Bichromicum
Sulphur
Nux Vomica
Red:
Aconitum Napellus
Mercurius Vivus
Nux Vomica
Stuck Together In The Morning:
Rhus Toxicodendron
Sties:
Ferrum Phosphoricum
Rhus Toxicodendron
Swollen:
Aconitum Napellus
Arsenicum Album
Kali Bichromicum
Lycopodium Clavatum
Mercurius Vivus
Nux Vomica
Rhus Toxicodendron
Swollen And Burning:
Euphrasia Officinalis*
Swollen Under Eyes:
Arsenicum Album
Twitching:
Belladonna
Worse:
Eye Symptoms Worse Outdoors:

Euphrasia Officinalis*

Face:

Circles:
Circles Around Eyes:
Nux Vomica

Color:
Blue Circles Under Eyes:
Lycopodium Clavatum
Flushed:
Gelsemium Sempervirens
Pulsatilla Nigricans
Flushed Face With Reddened Lips:
Belladonna
Pale:
Kali Bichromicum
Lycopodium Clavatum
Mercurius Vivus
Natrum Muriaticum
Nux Vomica
Rhus Toxicodendron
Phosphorus
Sulphur
Pale Face, Flushes Easily:
Ferrum Phosphoricum
Paler In The Evening:
Lycopodium Clavatum
Red:
Aconitum Napellus
Belladonna
Ferrum Phosphoricum
Red Cheeks:
Euphrasia Officinalis
Lycopodium Clavatum
Red Without Much Fever:
Sulphur
Yellow:
Gelsemium Sempervirens
Mercurius Vivus
Natrum Muriaticum
Sulphur

Yellow With Blue Circles Under The Eyes:
Hepar Sulphuris Calcareum
Yellow Around Nose And Mouth:
Nux Vomica

Hot:
Burning Face:
Sulphur
Hot And Heavy Face:
Gelsemium Sempervirens
Hot And Pale Face:
Calcarea Carbonica

Jaws:
Jaws Crack When Chewing:
Rhus Toxicodendron

Pain:
Ferrum Phosphoricum
Pain Better From Heat:
Pulsatilla Nigricans
Pain Extends To Ear On The Painful Side:
Nux Vomica
Pain One Side Of Face, Watery Nasal Discharge
From The Nostril On The Same Side:
Nux Vomica
Pain Right Half Of Face:
Belladonna
Pulsatilla Nigricans
Pain Worse Evening:
Rhus Toxicodendron
Pressing Pain Cheekbones And Bridge Of
Nose:
Kali Bichromicum

Sweat:
Sweats On Face:
Nux Vomica

Swollen Or Puffy
Puffy:
Calcarea Carbonica
Mercurius Vivus
Swollen:
Bryonia

Rhus Toxicodendron
Phosphorus
Swollen, One Side Of Face:
Nux Vomica
Swollen Upper Lip:
Lycopodium Clavatum
Tightness:
Forehead:
Pulsatilla Nigricans

Fever:

Fever, General:
Anas Barbarae
Fever Symptoms:
Doesn't Recover After The Fever:
Natrum Muriaticum
Fever Better From Sleep:
Eupatorium Perfoliatum
Fever Comes And Goes:
Rhus Toxicodendron
Fever From Drugging:
Nux Vomica
Fever Goes To Chest Or Liver To Produce Jaundice:
Eupatorium Perfoliatum
Fever With Convulsions Or Teething:
Belladonna
Fever With Hallucinations:
Belladonna
Fever With Seeing Ghosts, Insects, And
Black Animals:
Belladonna
Fever With No Other Symptoms:
Ferrum Phosphoricum*
Fever With No Thirst:
Belladonna*
Fever With Starting And Jumping:
Belladonna
Recurrent Fever With No Symptoms:
Ferrum Phosphoricum*
Chills:
Pulsatilla Nigricans
Chills Alternate With Fever:
Phosphorus
Rhus Toxicodendron
Chills Alternate With Burning Heat:
Arsenicum Album
Chills Alternate With Dry Heat With Profuse
Perspiration:
Hepar Sulphuris Calcareum

Chills Between Diarrhetic Stools:
　　Mercurius Vivus
Chills From The Slightest Breeze:
　　Hepar Sulphuris Calcareum
Chills Preceded By Thirst:
　　Eupatorium Perfoliatum
Chills Predominate The Fever:
　　Euphrasia Officinalis
　　Nux Vomica
Chills When Unwrapped:
　　Aconitum Napellus
Chills With Blue Fingernails:
　　Nux Vomica
Chills With Nausea And Vomiting:
　　Lycopodium Clavatum
Chills Worse Uncovered:
　　Nux Vomica
Cold Chills Pass Through Him:
　　Aconitum Napellus
Shivering/Shaking:
　　Shaking:
　　　　Eupatorium Perfoliatum
　　　　Gelsemium Sempervirens
　　Shivering:
　　　　Bryonia
　　　　Eupatorium Perfoliatum*
　　　　Phosphorus
　　　　Sulphur
　　　　Shivers After Drinking:
　　　　　　Nux Vomica
　　　　Shivers When Moved:
　　　　　　Nux Vomica
　　Trembling:
　　　　Kali Bichromicum
　　　　Trembling And Nausea From
　　　　Motion During Fever:
　　　　　　Eupatorium
　　　　Violent Spasms:
　　　　(Especially In The Morning):
　　　　　　Eupatorium Perfoliatum*

Time:
Chills In The Afternoon:
Pulsatilla Nigricans
Chills At 1:00 In The Afternoon:
Ferrum Phosphoricum
Chills In The Evening:
Hepar Sulphuris Calcareum
Chills 6:00 -7:00 In The Evening:
Hepar Sulphuris Calcareum
Chills In The Evening, Mostly On One Side:
Bryonia
Chills In The Morning:
Euphrasia Officinalis
Gelsemium Sempervirens
Chills In The Morning And When Rising:
Mercurius Vivus
Chills Worse 7:00-9:00 In The Morning:
Eupatorium Perfoliatum*
9:00 In The Morning To Noon:
Natrum Muriaticum
Between 9:00 And 11:00 In The Morning:
Natrum Muriaticum
Chilliness Same Time Each Day:
Gelsemium Sempervirens
Headache:
With Chill During Fever:
Natrum Muriaticum
Hot And Cold:
Alternately Cold And Hot:
Aconitum Napellus
Cold Hands And Feet With Fever:
Gelsemium Sempervirens
Head Burns, But Rest Of Body Cold:
Aconitum Napellus
Skin Hot And Dry:
Aconitum Napellus
Skin Hot To Touch:
Belladonna
Onset Of Fever (See Also Cause/Onset):
Early Stages Of Flu:

Aconitum Napellus
Sudden And Violent, After Chill:
Aconitum Napellus
Sudden Onset With High Fever:
Belladonna
Rapid Onset With Anxiety And Restlessness:
Arsenicum Album

Perspiration/Sweat:
Calcarea Carbonica
Rhus Toxicodendron
Sweats Easily And Profusely:
Allium Cepa
Sweats From Least Exercise:
Lycopodium Clavatum
Sweats Around Head, Neck, And Chest:
Calcarea Carbonica
Night Sweats:
Calcarea Carbonica
Euphrasia Officinalis
Rhus Toxicodendron
Sweats On Nape Of Neck And Back Of Head
At Night:
Sulphur
Debilitating Night Sweats:
Mercurius Vivus

Skin:
Red:
Sulphur
So Hot It Radiates Heat:
Belladonna

Time: (See Also Chills: Time):
Morning:
Comes On After Midnight With Thirst:
Mercurius Vivus
Highest Temperature Between Midnight And
3:00 In The Morning:
Arsenicum Album
Fever Peaks Every Third Day:
Eupatorium Perfoliatum
Fever Worse: Evening:

Rhus Toxicodendron
4:00-8:00 In The Evening:
        Lycopodium Clavatum
Night:
Worse At Night:
        Belladonna
Fever Peaks At 9:00 At Night:
        Aconitum Napellus

Food And Drink:

Aggravation:
Alcoholic Drinks Give Hay Fever:
Arsenicum Album
Beans:
Lycopodium Clavatum
Broccoli:
Lycopodium Clavatum
Cabbage:
Lycopodium Clavatum
Coffee:
Arsenicum Album
Cold Drinks:
Arsenicum Album
Eggs:
Sulphur
Fat:
Animal Fat Aggravates:
Nux Vomica
Ice Cream:
Arsenicum Album
Meat:
Kali Bichromicum
Nux Vomica
Milk:
Arsenicum Album
Calcarea Carbonica
Lycopodium Clavatum
Sulphur
Nuts:
Arsenicum Album
Onions:
Lycopodium Clavatum
Pastry:
Lycopodium Clavatum
Peas:
Lycopodium Clavatum
Reheated Food:
Lycopodium Clavatum

Rich Food:
>   Pulsatilla Nigricans

Salt:
>   Excess Salt:
>> Phosphorus

Sea Food:
>   Arsenicum Album

Sugar:
>   Arsenicum Album

Sweets:
>   Mercurius Vivus

Wheat:
>   Arsenicum Album

Wine:
>   Calcarea Carbonica

Appetite:

A Little Food Fills Up And Gives Gas:
>   Lycopodium Clavatum

Capricious, Changeable:
>   Lycopodium Clavatum
>   Pulsatilla Nigricans

Dislikes The Smell and Sight Of Food:
>   Arsenicum Album

Faddish About Food:
>   Phosphorus

Full With Little Food:
>   Nux Vomica

Hungry:
>   Mercurius Vivus
>   Excessive Appetite:
>> Sulphur
>   Increased Appetite:
>> Gelsemium Sempervirens
>   Hunger Between Meals:
>   Phosphorus

Hungry But Dislike Of Food:
>   Nux Vomica

No Appetite:
>   Arsenicum Album

Bryonia
Nux Vomica
Rhus Toxicodendron
No Appetite In The Morning But Snacks
During The Day:
Sulphur
Not Hungry For Breakfast:
Sulphur
Poor Appetite:
Arsenicum Album
Bryonia
Ferrum Phosphoricum
Hepar Sulphuris Calcareum
Lycopodium Clavatum
Nux Vomica
Ravenous:
Pulsatilla Nigricans
Ravenous Hunger With Attacks Of
Vomiting:
Sulphur
Small Or Little Amounts Of Food Fill Up Or Satisfy:
Gelsemium Sempervirens
Lycopodium Clavatum
Weak And Faint At 11:00 In The Morning, Needs
Something To Eat:
Sulphur

Aversion:
Acids:
Sulphur
Alcohol:
Sulphur
Beer:
Phosphorus
Cucumbers:
Allium Cepa
Boiled Foods:
Calcarea Carbonica
Bread:
Natrum Muriaticum

Butter:
>Arsenicum Album
>Calcarea Carbonica
>Ferrum Phosphoricum
>Mercurius Vivus

Coffee:
>Lycopodium Clavatum
>Mercurius Vivus
>Phosphorus

Cooked Food:
>Mercurius Vivus

Cooked Meat:
>Lycopodium Clavatum

Eggs:
>Sulphur

Fish:
>Phosphorus

Fat:
>Arsenicum Album
>Hepar Sulphuris Calcareum
>Natrum Muriaticum
>Mercurius Vivus
>Sulphur
>Pulsatilla Nigricans

Hot Food:
>Calcarea Carbonica

Meat:
>Arsenicum Album
>Calcarea Carbonica
>Ferrum Phosphoricum
>Kali Bichromicum
>Mercurius Vivus
>Phosphorus
>Sulphur

Milk:
>Pulsatilla Nigricans
>Sulphur

Plain Water:
>Sulphur

Pork:

Pulsatilla Nigricans
Rye Bread:
Lycopodium Clavatum
Sulphur
Salt:
Natrum Muriaticum
Sulphur
Slimy Food:
Natrum Muriaticum
Spicy Food:
Sulphur
Squash:
Sulphur
Sweets:
Sulphur
Tea:
Phosphorus
Warm Food:
Lycopodium Clavatum

Desires:
Acid Drinks:
Bryonia
Acid Food:
Hepar Sulphuris Calcareum
Sulphur
Alcohol:
Hepar Sulphuris Calcareum
Mercurius Vivus
Nux Vomica
Beer:
Kali Bichromicum
Butter:
Pulsatilla Nigricans
Chocolate:
Phosphorus
Coffee:
Bryonia
Nux Vomica
Creamy Foods:
Pulsatilla Nigricans

Eggs:
> Calcarea Carbonica

Fat:
> Arsenicum Album
> Nux Vomica
> Sulphur

Fish:
> Phosphorus

Hot Drinks:
> Arsenicum Album

Hot Meals:
> Lycopodium Clavatum

Ice Cream:
> Calcarea Carbonica
> Eupatorium Perfoliatum
> Phosphorus
> Pulsatilla Nigricans

Lemonade:
> Belladonna

Milk:
> Arsenicum Album
> Calcarea Carbonica
> Nux Vomica
> Phosphorus
> Cold Milk:
>> Phosphorus

Oysters:
> Rhus Toxicodendron

Peanut Butter:
> Pulsatilla Nigricans

Pickles:
> Arsenicum Album
> Ferrum Phosphoricum
> Sulphur

Raw Onions:
> Allium Cepa

Salt:
> Calcarea Carbonica
> Natrum Muriaticum
> Phosphorus

Sulphur
Stimulants:
Nux Vomica
Sour Food:
Calcarea Carbonica
Ferrum Phosphoricum
Spicy Food:
Hepar Sulphuris Calcareum
Nux Vomica
Phosphorus
Strong Tasting Food:
Hepar Sulphuris Calcareum
Sulphur
Starch:
Calcarea Carbonica
Sugar:
Lycopodium Clavatum
Sweets:
Arsenicum Album
Calcarea Carbonica
Kali Bichromicum
Lycopodium Clavatum
Sulphur
Tea:
Natrum Muriaticum
Vinegar:
Arsenicum Album
Ferrum Phosphoricum
Hepar Sulphuris Calcareum
Warm Drinks:
Arsenicum Album
Lycopodium Clavatum
Water:
Rhus Toxicodendron
Wine:
Bryonia
Mercurius Vivus
Taste: (See Also Mouth)
Tastes Bitter:
Arsenicum Album

Food Tastes Bitter Except Water:
Aconitum Napellus
Food Tastes Tasteless:
Bryonia
Food Tastes Too Sweet:
Bryonia
Rye Bread Tastes Bitter Or Sweet:
Mercurius Vivus

Thirst:

Allium Cepa
Belladonna
Kali Bichromicum
Lycopodium Clavatum
Natrum Muriaticum
Nux Vomica
Rhus Toxicodendron*
After Chills:
Eupatorium Perfoliatum
Beer:
Sulphur
Mercurius Vivus
Before Chill:
Pulsatilla Nigricans
Carbonated Drinks:
Phosphorus
Cold Drinks:
Calcarea Carbonica
Eupatorium Perfoliatum
Ferrum Phosphoricum
Hepar Sulphuris Calcareum
Kali Bichromicum
Mercurius Vivus
Natrum Muriaticum
Rhus Toxicodendron
Phosphorus
Cold Drinks Especially At Night:
Calcarea Carbonica
Cold Drinks, Which They Gulp:
Bryonia*
Cold Water:

Belladonna
Large Quantities Of Cold Water:
Aconitum Napellus
Belladonna
Bryonia
Eupatorium Perfoliatum
Lemonade:
Belladonna*
Milk:
Mercurius Vivus
Small Sips:
Arsenicum Album
Thirstless:
Belladonna
Gelsemium Sempervirens
Lycopodium Clavatum
Nux Vomica
Pulsatilla Nigricans

Generalities:

Behavior (See Also Cold Traits):
Bites People (Children):
Belladonna
Constantly Blowing Nose:
Kali Bichromicum*
Delirium:
Belladonna
Inability To Turn Over In Bed Without Sitting Up:
Nux Vomica
Fidgety:
Arsenicum Album
Phosphorus
Lie Still:
Wants To Lie Still:
Bryonia
Lethargic:
Calcarea Carbonica
Nervousness:
Belladonna
Nervous, Tense Before Thunderstorms:
Nux Vomica
Passive:
Calcarea Carbonica
Puts Feet Out Of Covers At Night:
Sulphur*
Quick Movements:
Arsenicum Album
Rapidly:
Does Everything Rapidly:
Nux Vomica
Restless:
Aconitum Napellus
Arsenicum Album
Restless, But Tries To Stay Still Because Movement Hurts:
Eupatorium Perfoliatum

Sits With Hands Flat On Knees, Shoulders Raised
To Support Chest/Breathing:
>Eupatorium Perfoliatum
Violent Behavior Of Children:
>Belladonna

Chilly (In General, See Also "Chills" Under "Fever"):
Aconitum Napellus
Arsenicum Album*
Calcarea Carbonica
Gelsemium Sempervirens
Lycopodium Clavatum
Begins In Stomach:
>Calcarea Carbonica
Can't Get Warm:
>Euphrasia Officinalis
Not Helped By Covering Up:
>Arsenicum Album*
>Natrum Muriaticum*
Chills Alternate With Heat:
>Nux Vomica
Chills And Shivering With Slightest
Movement:
>Nux Vomica
Chills At 2:00 In The Afternoon:
>Calcarea Carbonica
Chills Begin In Hands And Feet With Pain In
Limbs:
>Pulsatilla Nigricans
Increased Thirst After Chills:
>Eupatorium Perfoliatum
Wants Fresh Or Cool Air Even When Chilled:
>Pulsatilla Nigricans
Clothing:
Loosens Or Hates Tight Clothing:
>Calcarea Carbonica
>Eupatorium Perfoliatum
>Nux Vomica
>Around Abdomen:

Lycopodium Clavatum
Cold Traits: (See Also Behavior)
Colds Are Worse From Asthma:
Arsenicum Album
Cold Begins In Nose And Moves Down To Chest:
Arsenicum Album*
Bryonia*
Cold Begins In Nose And Moves To Larynx:
Euphrasia Officinalis*
Cold Begins In The Chest:
Phosphorus*
Cold Lingers:
Gelsemium Sempervirens*
Cold Reoccurs:
Arsenicum Album*
Calcarea Carbonica*
Sulphur*
Reoccurs With Periodicity:
Arsenicum Album*
Sulphur*
Cold Settles In Nose And Goes To Chest:
Lycopodium Clavatum*
Dry Cold Without Nasal Discharge:
Belladonna*
Early Stages Of Cold With Few Symptoms:
Ferrum Phosphoricum*
Sneezes At Every Change Of Weather:
Arsenicum Album
Symptoms Change Frequently:
Pulsatilla Nigricans*
Takes Cold A Lot:
Arsenicum Album
Takes Cold At Every Change Of Weather:
Calcarea Carbonica
Constipation:
Constipation Alternating With Diarrhea:
Sulphur
Constipation With Hard, Dark Feces:
Phosphorus
Constipation With No Desire For BM:

Nux Vomica

Diarrhea:
From:

Anticipation Of An Ordeal:
Gelsemium Sempervirens
Emotional Excitement:
Gelsemium Sempervirens

Stool:

Dark Brown:
Mercurius Vivus
Green:
Ferrum Phosphoricum
Mercurius Vivus
Involuntary Stool When Coughing:
Phosphorus
Loose And Burning:
Sulphur
Watery:
Ferrum Phosphoricum
Mercurius Vivus
Watery And Painless Diarrhea:
Phosphorus

When:

Morning:
Nux Vomica
Morning, Drives Out Of Bed:
Sulphur*

With:

Anus Sore:
Sulphur
Constipation:
Constipation Alternating With
Diarrhea:
Sulphur
Fever:
Ferrum Phosphoricum
Gas:
Sulphur
Rectal Itching:
Sulphur

Retching:
> Ferrum Phosphoricum

Worse Midnight To Morning:
> Ferrum Phosphoricum

Yellow Stool:
> Mercurius Vivus

Heart:

Heart Palpitations:
> Aconitum Napellus

Hot And Cold:

Feels Bad In A Warm Room, But Cannot Bear
The Cold:
> Mercurius Vivus

Muscles:

Jerking:
> Natrum Muriaticum

Trembling:
> Natrum Muriaticum
> Phosphorus

Twitching:
> Gelsemium Sempervirens
> Natrum Muriaticum

Pain:

Aching:
> Anas Barbarae
> Arsenicum Album

Aches Getting Out Of A Seat:
> Rhus Toxicodendron

Alternates From Left To Right:
> Allium Cepa

Better:

Better From Pressure:
> Bryonia

Bones:
> Eupatorium Perfoliatum

Bruised:
> Mercurius Vivus

Burning:

Allium Cepa
Burning Pain In Head, Back,
Extremities:
Arsenicum Album
Movement:
Can't Move Because Of Pain:
Eupatorium Perfoliatum
Moves:
Pain Moves From Place To Place:
Kali Bichromicum
Sharp And Burning Moving Pain:
Kali Bichromicum
Small Spots:
Kali Bichromicum
Speed:
Pain Appears Fast, Goes Slowly, Or Pain
Appears Slowly And Leaves Quickly:
Pulsatilla Nigricans
Tearing:
Bryonia
Rhus Toxicodendron

Perspiration:
Around Head:
Calcarea Carbonica*
From:
Eating:
Natrum Muriaticum
Taking Warm Drink:
Rhus Toxicodendron
Frequently:
Sulphur
Profusely:
Sulphur
Profusely Around 2:00 in the morning:
Bryonia
Profusely In The Morning:
Pulsatilla Nigricans
Profusely With Anxiety:
Aconitum Napellus

Smell Of Sweat:
>> Offensive:
>>> Mercurius Vivus
>> Sour:
>>> Bryonia
>>> Calcarea Carbonica
>>> Sulfur
> When:
>> At Night With No Relief:
>>> Hepar Sulphuris Calcareum
>> In Sleep:
>>> Calcarea Carbonica
> Where:
>> Around Head, Neck, Upper Body:
>>> Calcarea
>> On Covered Parts:
>>> Belladonna
>> On Upper Body Only:
>>> Euphrasia Officinalis

Senses:
> Acute:
>> Belladonna
> Over Sensitive:
>> Aconitum Napellus

Sensitive To:
> Chair Or Couch Feels Hard:
>> Lycopodium Clavatum
> Cold:
>> Belladonna
>> Calcarea Carbonica
>> Especially Around Ears And Neck:
>>> Calcarea Carbonica
> Cold Air:
>> Rhus Toxicodendron
> Cold Drafts:
>> Rhus Toxicodendron
> Disturbance:
>> Hepar Sulphuris Calcareum
> Drafts:

Arsenicum Album
Belladonna
Least Draft:
Nux Vomica
External Stimuli:
Phosphorus
Light:
Belladonna
Noise:
Belladonna
Hates Sound Of Wind:
Nux Vomica
Worse Listening To Music:
Aconitum Napellus
Odors:
Faints From Odors When Ill:
Nux Vomica
Open Air:
Sulphur
Pain:
Hepar Sulphuris Calcareum
Nux Vomica
Tobacco Smoke:
Tobacco Smoke Makes Nauseated And
Have Heart Palpitations:
Phosphorus
Touch:
Hepar Sulphuris Calcareum
Skin:
Bright Red:
Ear Canals, Anus, Nostrils May Be Bright Red:
Sulphur*
Dry:
Aconitum Napellus
Belladonna
Feels Hot But They Are Cold Inside:
Arsenicum Album
Itches:
Rhus Toxicodendron
Sulphur

Moist:
> Calcarea Carbonica

Oversensitive:
> Aconitum Napellus

Pale, Cold, Clammy:
> Arsenicum Album

Red:
> Belladonna*

So Hot It Radiates Heat:
> Belladonna*

Sidedness:

One Sided Complaints:
> Pulsatilla Nigricans

One Sided Chilliness Turns To One Sided Heat
Which Turns To One-Sided Sweat:
> Pulsatilla Nigricans

Right Sided:
> Belladonna
> Lycopodium Clavatum

Moves From Above Downwards:
> Lycopodium Clavatum

Moves From Right To Left:
> Lycopodium Clavatum

Urinary:

Urine Spills When Coughing:
> Natrum Muriaticum

Vascular:

Flushing And Throbbing Symptoms:
> Belladonna

Weakness/Fatigue:

Profound Weakness:
> Arsenicum Album
> Gelsemium Sempervirens*

Wants To Lie Down:
> Ferrum Phosphoricum

From:
> Least Exertion:

Calcarea Carbonica
Mercurius Vivus
Talking:
Talking Fatigues And Makes The Headache
Worse:
Sulphur
Tired Eyes, During The Day:
Euphrasia Officinalis

Head:

Better:
        Cold:
                Arsenicum Album
                Ferrum Phosphoricum
        Cold Weather:
                Lycopodium Clavatum
        Eating, After Eating:
                Arsenicum Album
                Lycopodium Clavatum
                Phosphorus
        Getting Up:
                Mercurius Vivus
        Lying Down:
                Natrum Muriaticum
                Lying Down With Head High:
                        Natrum Muriaticum
        Motion:
                Lycopodium Clavatum
                Mercurius Vivus
        Open Air:
                Kali Bichromicum
                Phosphorus
        Long Walk In Open Air:
                Rhus Toxicodendron
        Sleep:
                Gelsemium Sempervirens
        Vomiting:
                Ferrum Phosphoricum
                Mercurius Vivus
                Natrum Muriaticum
        Warm Room:
                Sulphur
        Wrapping Head Tightly:
                Belladonna

Dry:
        Belladonna

Headache:
        Allium Cepa

Eupatorium Perfoliatum
When Chilled:
> Eupatorium Perfoliatum

Coughing:
> Bryonia

With Burning Tears On Affected Side:
> Pulsatilla Nigricans

Cold Hands And Feet:
> Calcarea Carbonica

Dullness Of Mind:
> Rhus Toxicodendron

Head Tender To The Touch:
> Mercurius Vivus

Loss Of Hair:
> Mercurius Vivus

With Nausea:
> In Right Temple:
>> Gelsemium Sempervirens
> Nausea And Vomiting:
>> Kali Bichromicum
>> Natrum Muriaticum

Scalp Sore: Kali Bichromicum
> Nux Vomica

Roots Of Hair Sore:
> Nux Vomica

Skin Of Forehead Feels Tight:
> Phosphorus

Strong Pulse Of Arteries:
> Belladonna
> Gelsemium Sempervirens

Vision Disturbances:
> Dazzling In Front Of Eyes:
>> Euphrasia Officinalis
> Visual Impairment Or Blindness:
>> Kali Bichromicum

Vomiting:
> Ferrum Phosphoricum
> Mercurius Vivus

Headache Causes:
> Coughing:

Bryonia
Mercurius Vivus
Phosphorus
Discharge:
Headache Returns When Thick
Yellow Discharge Returns:
Lycopodium Clavatum
Hunger:
Phosphorus
Sulphur
Indigestion:
Pulsatilla Nigricans
Overwork:
Pulsatilla Nigricans
One Sided After Overwork:
Nux Vomica
Rebound Headache After Week's Work:
Sulphur
Type Of Headache:
Congestive Headache:
Belladonna
Pressure:
Aconitum Napellus
Pressure Top Of Head:
Kali Bichromicum
Severe:
Belladonna
Bryonia
Stuffy:
Eupatorium Perfoliatum
Stuffy With Lots Of Discharge:
Euphrasia Officinalis
Location:
Above Right Eye And Extending To Nose:
Calcarea Carbonica
Back Of Head (Occiput):
Belladonna
Gelsemium Sempervirens
Nux Vomica
Back To Front Of Head, When Stooping:

Ferrum Phosphoricum
Frontal:
Nux Vomica
Forehead:
Allium Cepa
Belladonna
Bryonia
Natrum Muriaticum
Forehead, Aching And Shooting
Pain:
Bryonia
Forehead, with Nasal Congestion:
Allium Cepa*
Neck To Eyes And Forehead:
Gelsemium Sempervirens
Over Eyebrows:
Kali Bichromicum
Side:
One Sided:
Natrum Muriaticum
Left Sided With Dizziness:
Eupatorium Perfoliatum
Right Sided:
Belladonna
Rhus Toxicodendron
Temples:
Belladonna
Pulsatilla Nigricans
Right Temple:
Allium Cepa
Temples And Forehead, Shooting
Pain:
Euphrasia Officinalis
Temples And Forehead, Throbbing
Pain:
Ferrum Phosphoricum
Quality Of Pain:
Bursting:
Bryonia
Euphrasia Officinalis

Gelsemium Sempervirens
Natrum Muriaticum
Sulphur
Pounding:
Gelsemium Sempervirens
Ringing:
Hepar Sulphuris Calcareum
Severe:
Belladonna*
Sharp:
Ferrum Phosphoricum
Shooting:
Euphrasia Officinalis
Splitting:
Bryonia
Throbbing:
Anas Barbarae
Calcarea Carbonica
Phosphorus
Sulphur
Starts With Nasal Discharge, Then
Discharge Stops and Throbbing
Headache Begins:
Belladonna*
Throbs With Movement:
Belladonna*
Violent:
Gelsemium Sempervirens
Hot:
Aconitum Napellus
Gelsemium Sempervirens
With Cold Extremities:
Belladonna
With Pale Face:
Calcarea Carbonica
Worse Movement:
Aconitum Napellus
Tightness, Forehead:
Pulsatilla Nigricans*
Vertigo (Dizziness):

Gelsemium Sempervirens
Lycopodium Clavatum
In The Evening:
    Arsenicum Album
    Hepar Sulphuris Calcareum
In The Morning:
    Kali Bichromicum
    Rhus Toxicodendron
    Phosphorus
In Open Air:
    Nux Vomica
    Pulsatilla Nigricans
Makes Them Fall Forward And To The Left:
    Natrum Muriaticum
Makes Them Fall To The Left Side Or Backwards:
    Belladonna
Makes Them Stager To The Right:
    Rhus Toxicodendron
When:
    Ascending:
        Calcarea Carbonica
        Sulphur
    Coughing:
        Nux Vomica
    Eating:
        After Eating:
            Sulphur
    Exercising In Open Air:
        Sulphur
    Eyes, Using Eyes:
        Pulsatilla Nigricans
    Lying Down:
        Pulsatilla Nigricans
    Lying On Back:
        Mercurius Vivus
    Medication:
        After Medication:
            Nux Vomica
    Moving Eyes:
        Hepar Sulphuris Calcareum

Moving Head:
> Aconitum Napellus
> Calcarea Carbonica
> Hepar Sulphuris Calcareum

When Rising:
> Aconitum Napellus

Rising From Seat Or Bed:
> Mercurius Vivus
> Sulphur

Shutting Eyes:
> Arsenicum Album

Sitting:
> Pulsatilla Nigricans

Sneezing:
> Nux Vomica

Stooping:
> Bryonia
> Kali Bichromicum
> Nux Vomica
> Pulsatilla Nigricans

Walking:
> Nux Vomica

With Loss Of Consciousness:
> Nux Vomica

Worse (Head Symptoms Worse):

Anger:
> Nux Vomica

Coughing:
> Hepar Sulphuris Calcareum
> Mercurius Vivus
> Natrum Muriaticum
> Phosphorus
> Rhus Toxicodendron
> Sulphur

Drinking:
> Mercurius Vivus

Eating:
> Mercurius Vivus

Night Or Early Morning:
> Calcarea Carbonica

Not Eating:
> Nux Vomica

Light:
> Bryonia
> Gelsemium Sempervirens
> Kali Bichromicum

Lying Down:
> Lycopodium Clavatum

Morning:
> Kali Bichromicum
> Natrum Muriaticum
> Begins In The Morning And Gets Worse
> Afternoon And Evening:
>> Eupatorium Perfoliatum
>> Gelsemium Sempervirens

Movement:
> Bryonia
> Gelsemium Sempervirens
> Hepar Sulphuris Calcareum
> Phosphorus

Night:
> Kali Bichromicum
> Mercurius Vivus

Nasal Discharge:
> The Less The Nasal Discharge The
> Worse The Headache:
>> Bryonia
> Throbbing Headache alternating with Nasal
> Discharge:
>> Belladonna*

Noise:
> Bryonia
> Kali Bichromicum

Outdoors:
> Mercurius Vivus
> Nux Vomica
> Sulphur

Pale Face:
> Natrum Muriaticum

Sitting Up:

Aconitum Napellus
Sleeping:
Mercurius Vivus
Standing:
Rhus Toxicodendron
Stooping:
Aconitum Napellus
Bryonia
Calcarea Carbonica
Sweating:
Eupatorium Perfoliatum
Ferrum Phosphoricum
Hepar Sulphuris Calcareum
Kali Bichromicum
Lycopodium Clavatum
Cold Sweat:
Cold Sweat After Least Exercise:
Hepar Sulphuris Calcareum
On The Head At Night:
Hepar Sulphuris Calcareum
Talking:
Pressure On The Head Is Worse Talking:
Aconitum Napellus
Time:
5:00 In The Afternoon:
Ferrum Phosphoricum
4:00-8:00 In The Evening:
Lycopodium Clavatum
9:00 In The Morning:
Kali Bichromicum
10:00-11:00 In The Morning Headache
Starts:
Natrum Muriaticum
Top Of The Head:
Lycopodium Clavatum
Waking Up:
Mercurius Vivus
Walking:
Kali Bichromicum
Nux Vomica

Rhus Toxicodendron

Larynx:

Cold Centers On The Larynx:
Rhus Toxicodendron
Hoarseness/Laryngitis:
Aconitum Napellus
Anas Barbarae
Arsenicum Album
Bryonia
Ferrum Phosphoricum
Gelsemium Sempervirens
Natrum Muriaticum
Rhus Toxicodendron
Better Using The Voice:
Rhus Toxicodendron
Comes And Goes:
Pulsatilla Nigricans
Early Stages:
Allium Cepa
Hoarse In The Morning:
Euphrasia Officinalis
Hoarseness In Dry Cold Wind:
Hepar Sulphuris Calcareum
Painful Hoarseness Or Roughness:
Nux Vomica
Painless Hoarseness:
Calcarea Carbonica*
Rhus Toxicodendron
Severe Laryngitis:
Belladonna
Sudden Hoarseness:
Belladonna
Irritated:
Euphrasia Officinalis
Worse:
Worse In The Morning:
Eupatorium Perfoliatum
Worse In The Evening:
Kali Bichromicum
Phosphorus

Worse Talking And Coughing:
> Hepar Sulphuris Calcareum

Mucus/Phlegm:
Bryonia
Euphrasia Officinalis
Phosphorus
Hawks Up Mucus:
> Euphrasia Officinalis

Lots Of Mucus:
> Calcarea Carbonica

Pain:
Aches When Breathing In:
> Aconitum Napellus
> Burning Pain:
> Arsenicum Album

Pain When Coughing:
> Allium Cepa
> Nux Vomica

Sore Larynx:
> Belladonna

When Swallowing:
> Hepar Sulphuris Calcareum

Sensations:
Burning Pain In Larynx:
> Rhus Toxicodendron

Burning And Tickling In Larynx With Hoarseness:
> Mercurius Vivus

Burning And Pricking In Larynx:
> Aconitum Napellus

Dry Larynx:
> Belladonna

Choking, Wakes 2:00 in the morning With A
Sensation Of Choking:
> Euphrasia Officinalis

Irritated:
> Euphrasia Officinalis
> Ferrum Phosphoricum

Spasms In Larynx, Feels Like Suffocating:
> Nux Vomica

Tickling In Windpipe:

Ferrum Phosphoricum
Ulcers:
Calcarea Carbonica
Voice:
Weak:
Gelsemium Sempervirens
Weak And Dull:
Lycopodium Clavatum

Lips:

Bleeding:
Bryonia
Blisters:
Hepar Sulphuris Calcareum
Fever Blisters:
Natrum Muriaticum*
Chapped:
Natrum Muriaticum
Pulsatilla Nigricans
Lower Lip Chapped:
Kali Bichromicum
Color:
Blackish:
Mercurius Vivus
Red:
Belladonna
Sulphur
Cracked:
Bryonia
Calcarea Carbonica
Natrum Muriaticum
Phosphorus
Rhus Toxicodendron
Lower Lip:
Kali Bichromicum
Crack In Center Of Lower Lip:
Phosphorus
Pulsatilla Nigricans
Dry:
Bryonia
Ferrum Phosphoricum
Gelsemium Sempervirens
Mercurius Vivus
Natrum Muriaticum
Rhus Toxicodendron
Sulfur
Hot:
Gelsemium Sempervirens

Licks Lips:
>Pulsatilla Nigricans

Pain:
>Top Of Lip Sore:
>>Allium Cepa

Peeling Lips:
>Pulsatilla Nigricans

Rough:
>Sulphur
>Mercurius Vivus

Scabs:
>Mercurius Vivus

Swollen:
>Lower Lip Swollen:
>>Kali Bichromicum

Ulcers:
>Mercurius Vivus

Mind:

Abusive:
Hepar Sulphuris Calcareum`

Anger:
Mercurius Vivus

Anger Alternating With Apathy:
Phosphorus
Nux Vomica

Furious Over Small Matters
Hepar Sulphuris Calcareum

Gets Angry Quickly And Quickly Remorseful:
Phosphorus

Wakes Up Angry Or Cross:
Lycopodium Clavatum

Anxiety (See Also Fears):
Aconitum Napellus
Arsenicum Album
Bryonia
Eupatorium Perfoliatum
Rhus Toxicodendron

About What:
Being Left Alone:
Arsenicum Album
Business:
Bryonia
Contagion:
Arsenicum Album
Death:
Arsenicum Album*
Germs:
Arsenicum Album
Health:
Arsenicum Album*
Home:
Calcarea Carbonica
Safety:
Calcarea Carbonica
Security:
Calcarea Carbonica

Nervous Anxiety:
Belladonna

Company:
Company Aggravates:
Avoids People:
Kali Bichromicum
Desires solitude:
Natrum Muriaticum
Rhus Toxicodendron
Wants to be left alone:
Bryonia
Gelsemium Sempervirens
Company Ameliorates:
Aconitum Napellus
Phosphorus*
Pulsatilla Nigricans*

Complains Constantly:
Hepar Sulphuris Calcareum

Comprehension:
Cloudy:
Rhus Toxicodendron
Slow:
Rhus Toxicodendron

Concentration:
Cannot Follow One Idea for a long time:
Gelsemium Sempervirens
Unable To Concentrate:
Ferrum Phos
Phosphorus*

Confusion:
Euphrasia

Consolation:
Consolation Makes Them Worse:
Natrum Muriaticum
Resents Consolation:
Nux Vomica
Sympathy Annoys:
Natrum Muriaticum

Crying:
Better from crying:

Pulsatilla Nigricans
Depression/Sadness:
Eupatorium Perfoliatum
Ferrum Phosphoricum
Hepar Sulphuris Calcareum
Natrum Muriaticum
At Twilight:
Rhus Toxicodendron
In Evening:
Hepar Sulphuris Calcareum
Despairing:
Lycopodium Clavatum
Despair About Never Recovering:
Arsenicum Album
Fear (See Also Anxiety):
Aconitum Napellus
Easily Frightened:
Phosphorus
Fearful But Can Be Bossy:
Lycopodium Clavatum
Fear Worse At Night:
Arsenicum Album
Of What:
Being Alone:
Lycopodium Clavatum
Claustrophobia:
Aconitum Napellus
Contagious Disease:
Anas Barbarae
Crowds:
Aconitum Napellus
Dark:
Phosphorus
Death:
Pulsatilla Nigricans
Disease:
Phosphorus
Earthquakes:
Aconitum Napellus
Falling:

Gelsemium Sempervirens
Having Hair Cut:
Aconitum Napellus
Heights:
Calcarea Carbonica
Flying:
Aconitum Napellus
Calcarea Carbonica
Germs:
Arsenicum Album
Pulsatilla Nigricans
Ghosts:
Phosphorus
Noise:
Calcarea Carbonica
Spiders:
Phosphorus
The Future:
Aconitum Napellus
Sulphur
Thunderstorms:
Phosphorus
Wrong:
Anything Going Wrong:
Arsenicum Album

Feels As Though He Might Die:
Aconitum Napellus
Hopeless:
Arsenicum Album
Hypersensitive:
Arsenicum Album*
Hepar Sulphuris Calcareum*
To Movement:
Nux Vomica
To Noise:
Nux Vomica
To Odors:
Nux Vomica
To Pain:
Nux Vomica

Irritable:
    Arsenicum Album
    Bryonia*
    Ferrum Phos
    Gelsemium Sempervirens
    Hepar Sulphuris Calcareum
    Nux Vomica*
    Frustrated In Little Things:
        Nux Vomica
    When Sick:
        Pulsatilla Nigricans

Lump In Throat On Emotional Occasions:
    Lycopodium Clavatum

Memory Weak (Forgetful):
    Calcarea Carbonica
    Ferrum Phos
    Gelsemium Sempervirens
    Hepar Sulphuris Calcareum
    Kali Bichromicum
    Lycopodium Clavatum
    Phosphorus*
    Sulphur
    Forgets names Of People, Streets, and Places:
        Mercurius Vivus
    Forgets What He Started To Do:
        Rhus Toxicodendron
    Forgets Words and Localities:
        Hepar Sulphuris Calcareum

Perseverance/Follow Through:
Lack of follow through:
    Phosphorus*
    Sulphur

Philosophical Ideas:
    Sulphur*

Religious Ideas:
    Sulphur*

Restless:
    Arsenicum Album
    Belladonna
    Eupatorium Perfoliatum

Mercurius Vivus
Rhus Toxicodendron
Restless especially at Night:
    Rhus Toxicodendron

Self-Confidence:
Low:
Rhus Toxicodendron

Suspicious:
Mercurius Vivus

Sympathy:
Better From Sympathy:
    Pulsatilla Nigricans*

Tension:
Nux Vomica

Touched:
Doesn't Want To Be Touched:
Nux Vomica

Traits:
Affectionate:
    Phosphorus
Apathetic:
    Gelsemium Sempervirens
    Apathy Alternating With Anger:
        Phosphorus
    Apathetic Regarding Illness:
        Gelsemium Sempervirens
Argumentative:
    Sulphur
Artistic:
    Phosphorus
Changeable:
    Pulsatilla Nigricans*
Clingy:
    Pulsatilla Nigricans
Critical:
    Nux Vomica
Dull and Listless/Aversion To Work:
    Eupatorium Perfoliatum
    Gelsemium Sempervirens
    Kali Bichromicum

Easily Offended:
>Nux Vomica

Emotional:
>Pulsatilla Nigricans

Equates Physical Weakness with Moral Deficiency:
>Lycopodium Clavatum*

Friendly:
>Phosphorus

Fussy and Tidy:
>Arsenicum Album*
>Nux Vomica

Happy:
>Natrum Muriaticum

Holds Grudges:
>Lycopodium Clavatum

In a Hurry:

Always In a Hurry:
>Lycopodium Clavatum

Independent:
>Calcarea Carbonica

Indecisive:
>Pulsatilla Nigricans

Mechanical Ability:
>Sulphur*

Mild Disposition:
>Pulsatilla Nigricans

Mirthful:
>Ferrum Phosphoricum

Moody:
>Pulsatilla Nigricans

Oversensitive:
>Nux Vomica

Philosophical, Abstract Thought:
>Sulphur*

Questions Everything:
>Hepar Sulphuris Calcareum

Resentful:
>Natrum Muriaticum

Selfish:
>Sulfur

Self-Pitying or Irritable When Sick:
        Pulsatilla Nigricans
Sensitive:
        Natrum Muriaticum
        Pulsatilla Nigricans
Shy:
        Pulsatilla Nigricans
Slow Answering Questions:
        Mercurius Vivus
Speculative:
        Sulphur
Sweet Natured:
        Pulsatilla Nigricans
Sympathetic:
        Phosphorus
Talk:
        Does not like to Talk:
                Euphrasia Officinalis
        Talkative:
                Ferrum Phosphoricum
        Talks In Obsessive Detail:
                Kali Bichromicum
Tidy, Neat:
        Arsenicum Album*
Unselfish:
        Sulphur
Untidy:
        Sulphur*
Weeps Easily:
        Pulsatilla Nigricans
Whiny:
        Pulsatilla Nigricans
Worried:
        Rhus Toxicodendron
Wants To Go Home:
Says They Want To Go Home:
        Bryonia*

Writing:
Spells Words Wrong Or Uses Words The Wrong
Way:

Lycopodium Clavatum
Drops Letters Out Of Words:
Lycopodium Clavatum
Omission of Words Or Syllables While Writing:
Nux Vomica

Mouth:

Breath:
Bad Breath:
Nux Vomica
Fetid Breath:
Gelsemium Sempervirens
Foul Breath:
Mercurius Vivus
Corners Of Mouth Sore:
Eupatorium Perfoliatum
Dry:
Aconitum Napellus
Arsenicum Album
Bryonia
Calcarea Carbonica
Kali Bichromicum
Nux Vomica
Rhus Toxicodendron
Pulsatilla Nigricans
Dry With No Thirst:
Lycopodium Clavatum
Gums:
Bleeding:
Phosphorus
Red:
Belladonna
Hot:
Ferrum Phosphoricum
Hot, Dry Mouth:
Belladonna
Sulphur
Jaws:
Jaws Crackle While Chewing:
Rhus Toxicodendron
Salivation:
Drools On Pillow:
Mercurius Vivus*
Increased Salivation:
Hepar Sulphuris Calcareum

        Kali Bichromicum
        Mercurius Vivus
Ropy, Stringy Saliva:
        Mercurius Vivus*
Saliva Tastes Sour, Salty, Sweet:
        Phosphorus
Too Much Saliva Or Dryness Of Mouth:
        Phosphorus

Taste:
Acid:
        Nux Vomica
Bad:
        Mercurius Vivus
Bitter:
        Nux Vomica
        Pulsatilla Nigricans
Metallic:
        Mercurius Vivus
        Nux Vomica
Putrid Taste:
        Gelsemium Sempervirens
Salty:
        Mercurius Vivus
        Nux Vomica
        Pulsatilla Nigricans
Sweet:
        Nux Vomica
Unpleasant Taste:
        Calcarea Carbonica
        Gelsemium Sempervirens
Loss Of Taste:
        Arsenicum Album
        Pulsatilla Nigricans

Teeth:
Teeth Ache With Hot Or Cold Fluids, Better
Rubbing Cheek On That Side:
        Mercurius Vivus

Ulcers/Cold Sores:
Ulcers:
        Arsenicum Album

Calcarea Carbonica
Hepar Sulphuris Calcareum
Mercurius Vivus*
Natrum Muriaticum*
Nux Vomica
Cold Sores:
Hepar Sulphuris Calcareum

Neck:

Carotids:
>Pulsing Carotids:
>>Belladonna*
>>Hepar Sulphuris Calcareum

Cracking:
>When Moving:
>>Pulsatilla Nigricans

Glandular Swelling And Pain:
>Pain:
>>Burning Or Stinging Pain In Lymph Nodes:
>>>Calcarea Carbonica
>>Painful Mastoid Gland:
>>>Gelsemium Sempervirens
>>>Nux Vomica
>>>Rhus Toxicodendron
>>Pain In Glands When Swallowing:
>>>Nux Vomica

>Swelling:
>>Belladonna
>>Calcarea Carbonica*
>>Kali Bichromicum
>>Lycopodium Clavatum
>>Mercurius Vivus
>>Rhus Toxicodendron
>>Phosphorus
>>Sulphur
>>Swollen Parotid Glands:
>>>Kali Bichromicum
>>>Painful And Swollen Parotid

>Glands:
>>Ferrum Phosphoricum
>>Hard Swelling Of Left Parotid
>>Gland:
>>>Kali Bichromicum
>>Swelling Of Right Parotid Gland
>>With Stinging Pain:
>>>Mercurius Vivus
>>Swollen Salivary Glands:

Mercurius Vivus

Stiff:

Aconitum Napellus
Anas Barbarae
Belladonna
Ferrum Phosphoricum
Nux Vomica
Rhus Toxicodendron
Sulphur
Stiff When Bending Forward:
    Kali Bichromicum
Stiff Left Side Of Neck:
    Lycopodium Clavatum
Stiff Nape:
    Belladonna
    Phosphorus

Rigid Nape Of Neck:

Nux Vomica
Pulsatilla Nigricans

Pain:

Bryonia
Better From Heat:
    Bryonia
Bruised Pain:
    Mercurius Vivus
Burning Pain Nape And Back Of Neck:
    Mercurius Vivus
Dull Ache:
    Gelsemium Sempervirens
    Natrum Muriaticum
Nape Of Neck:
    Allium Cepa
    Bryonia
Shooting Pain In Neck:
    Hepar Sulphuris Calcareum
    Pulsatilla Nigricans
Throbbing Pain In Nape Of Neck:
    Eupatorium Perfoliatum

Painful Stiffness:

Natrum Muriaticum

Nux Vomica
Painful Stiffness Back Of Neck:
>Bryonia

Swelling:

Belladonna
Swelling In Nape:
>Belladonna
Swelling Of Neck, Painful To Touch:
>Hepar Sulphuris Calcareum

Tension In Neck:

Natrum Muriaticum
Nux Vomica

Nose:
Blisters:
Natrum Muriaticum
Blocked:
Bryonia
Kali Bichromicum
Pulsatilla Nigricans
Blocked At Night:
Euphrasia Officinalis
Sulphur
Blocked During Sleep:
Calcarea Carbonica
Blocked At Night, Making Them Mouth
Breathe:
Lycopodium Clavatum
Blocked At Night, Runs During The Day:
Nux Vomica
Blocked Off and On:
Pulsatilla
Blows Nose Constantly:
Kali Bichromicum*
Burns And Itches:
Sulphur
Cold:
Tip Of Nose Cold:
Nux Vomica
Color Of Nose:
Red:
Belladonna
Red Nasal Membranes:
Belladonna
Red, Shiny, Sore:
Phosphorus
Tip Of Nose Red And Shiny:
Sulphur
Discharge:
Color Of Discharge:
Green:
Rhus Toxicodendron
Thick Green:

Pulsatilla Nigricans*
Tough Green Mucus:
Kali Bichromicum*
Mercurius Vivus
Greenish Yellow:
Kali Bichromicum*
Mercurius Vivus
White:
Natrum Muriaticum
Like Egg White:
Natrum Muriaticum
Yellow:
Calcarea Carbonica
Hepar Sulphuris Calcareum
Kali Bichromicum*
Sulphur
Yellow, Thick:
Rhus Toxicodendron*
Pulsatilla Nigricans*
Yellow, Thick, Chronic
Lycopodium Clavatum
Pulsatilla Nigricans*
Discharge Characteristics:
Alternately Stuffed Or Blocked And
Runny:
Nux Vomica
Phosphorus
Begins In Nose And Goes Down To
Throat:
Arsenicum Album
Better:
Cold Air
Nux Vomica
Clear Outside, Stuffed Up Or Bloody
Discharge Inside:
Pulsatilla Nigricans
Runs In Open Air, Stuffed Up Indoors:
Pulsatilla Nigricans (Opposite Of
Nux Vomica)

Runs In Warm Room And Stuffed Up Outdoors:
>> Arsenicum Album
>> Nux Vomica
>> Phosphorus

Shifts From Side To Side:
>> Allium Cepa
>> Phosphorus
>> Pulsatilla Nigricans

Starts At Left And Moves To Right:
>> Allium Cepa

Stops And Is Replaced By Throbbing Headache And High Fever:
>> Belladonna

Stops In Open Air And Starts In Warm Room:
>> Allium Cepa

Stuffed At Night And Indoors, Runs In Open Air:
>> Pulsatilla Nigricans

Worse:
> At Night:
>> Ferrum Phosphoricum
>> Pulsatilla Nigricans
> During Sleep:
>> Calcarea Carbonica
> Cold And Open Air:
>> Kali Bichromicum

Nosebleeds/Bloody Discharge:
> Nosebleeds:
>> Belladonna
>> Calcarea Carbonica
>> Euphrasia Officinalis
>> Bright Red Blood:
>>> Aconitum Napellus
>>> Ferrum Phosphoricum*
>> Clotted Black Blood:
>>> Mercurius Vivus
>>> Nux Vomica
>> Dark Blood:

                    Rhus Toxicodendron
                    Ferrum Phosphoricum
            Hot Blood:
                    Belladonna
        Blood In Nasal Discharge:
                    Euphrasia Officinalis
                    Ferrum Phosphoricum
                    Phosphorus
                    Pulsatilla Nigricans
                    Sulphur
    When:
            At Night:
                    Ferrum Phosphoricum
                    Rhus Toxicodendron
            In The Morning With Vertigo:
                    Sulphur
            When Hawking Mucus:
                    Rhus Toxicodendron
            When Stooping:
                    Rhus Toxicodendron
Quality Of Discharge:
    Acrid:
            Sulphur
    Bland:
            Euphrasia Officinalis
            Pulsatilla Nigricans
    Burning:
            Allium Cepa*
            Gelsemium Sempervirens
            Sulphur
            Burns Nose And Upper Lip:
                    Arsenicum Album
    Clear:
            Clear, Followed By Thick:
                    Anas Barbarae
            Clear Hot Water:
                    Aconitum Napellus
    Crusty:
            Bryonia
            Lycopodium Clavatum

Yellow Crusts Outside Nose:
Calcarea Carbonica
Profuse/Lots:
Aconitum Napellus
Allium Cepa
Hepar Sulphuris Calcareum
Natrum Muriaticum
Pulsatilla Nigricans
Profuse Discharge And Then
Stopped Up:
Natrum Muriaticum
Sticks Like Glue:
Kali Bichromicum
Thick:
Anas Barbarae
Calcarea Carbonica
Hepar Sulphuris Calcareum
Kali Bichromicum*
Natrum Muriaticum
Rhus Toxicodendron
Pulsatilla Nigricans*
Sulphur
Thin, Scanty:
Aconitum Napellus
Arsenicum Album
Belladonna
Thin, Watery, Stuffed Up At The
Same Time:
Arsenicum Album
Gelsemium Sempervirens
Tough Elastic Plugs In Nose:
Kali Bichromicum
Watery:
Aconitum Napellus
Allium Cepa
Arsenicum Album
Euphrasia Officinalis
Eupatorium Perfoliatum
Gelsemium Sempervirens
Hepar Sulphuris Calcareum

Natrum Muriaticum*

Dry Nose:
Belladonna*
Dry And Hot:
Gelsemium Sempervirens

Itches:
Mercurius Vivus
Nux Vomica
Burns And Itches:
Sulphur

Fanlike Movement Of Nose:
Lycopodium Clavatum

Food And Drink Regurgitate Through The Nose:
Lycopodium Clavatum

Fullness Root Of Nose:
Gelsemium Sempervirens

Inflamed:
Pulsatilla Nigricans

Pain:
Burns:
Allium Cepa
Nostrils Sore/Raw/Irritated
Calcarea Carbonica
Gelsemium Sempervirens
Mercurius Vivus
Tip Of Nose Red, Sore, Ulcerated:
Rhus Toxicodendron
Painful Dryness:
Phosphorus
Root Of Nose, Better By Pressure:
Kali Bichromicum
When Wiping Nose:
Allium Cepa

Pressure:
Pressure In Sinus And Root Of Nose:
Kali Bichromicum

Running:
Mercurius Vivus
Natrum Muriaticum

Pulsatilla Nigricans
Running Nose With Pain In Forehead:
Bryonia
Scabs In Nose:
Phosphorus
Sulphur
Sense Of Smell:
Absent/Dull:
Calcarea Carbonica
Hepar Sulphuris Calcareum
Phosphorus
Pulsatilla Nigricans
Sulphur
Acute/Sensitive:
Aconitum Napellus
Arsenicum Album
Belladonna
Calcarea Carbonica
Hepar Sulphuris Calcareum
Nux Vomica
Sulphur
Sensitive To Odor Of Peach Skins And
Flowers:
Allium Cepa
Sensitive To Odors Of Perfume Or
Tobacco:
Nux Vomica
Smells Foul Odor In Nose:
Belladonna
Sinus Congestion:
Hepar Sulphuris Calcareum
Pulsatilla Nigricans
Sneezing:
Gelsemium Sempervirens
Rhus Toxicodendron
Constant:
Allium Cepa
Sulphur
At Early Evening:
Gelsemium Sempervirens

Followed By Tingling And Fullness Of Nose:
   Gelsemium Sempervirens
Frequent:
      Belladonna
      Frequent And Painful:
         Arsenicum Album
      Frequent With Clear Mucus:
         Mercurius Vivus
      From Change In Temperature:
         Arsenicum Album
      From The Least Exposure To Cold Air:
         Hepar Sulphuris Calcareum
Lots Of Sneezing:
      Aconitum Napellus
      Eupatorium Perfoliatum
      Natrum Muriaticum
      Nux Vomica
      Lots, With No Relief:
         Arsenicum Album
Not Sneezing:
      Aconitum Napellus
Violent:
      Kali Bichromicum
With Pain In Head And Nape Of Neck:
      Calcarea Carbonica
Worse In Open Air:
      Kali Bichromicum

Stuffy:
      Aconitum Napellus
      Anas Barbarae
      Bryonia
      Gelsemium Sempervirens
      Mercurius Vivus
      Better Cold Air:
         Kali Bichromicum
      Dry And Stuffy:
         Kali Bichromicum
         Natrum Muriaticum
         Nux Vomica
         Rhus Toxicodendron

First Stage:
>Ferrum Phosphoricum

Stuffy At Night, Copious During The Morning:
>Pulsatilla Nigricans

Stuffiness Lingers:
>Calcarea Carbonica

Old Chronic Nasal Stuffiness:
>Arsenicum Album

Stuffy Noses In Children:
>Kali Bichromicum

Worse:
>In Open Air:
>>Kali Bichromicum

Swollen:
>Belladonna
>Bryonia
>Hepar Sulphuris Calcareum
>Natrum Muriaticum
>Rhus Toxicodendron
>Red, Swollen, Shining:
>>Mercurius Vivus
>With Pain:
>>Mercurius Vivus

Tickling In One Spot:
>Arsenicum Album

Tingling:
>Allium Cepa

Ulcers:
>Mercurius Vivus

Sensations:

Back:

Feels Bruised:
 Aconitum Napellus
 Nux Vomica
 Small Of Back Feels Bruised:
  Nux Vomica
Weight And Heaviness:
 Eupatorium Perfoliatum

Body:

Feels Too Heavy To Move:
 Gelsemium Sempervirens
Pains Like Electric Shock:
 Natrum Muriaticum
Waves Of Heat Along Spine:
 Gelsemium Sempervirens

Chest:

Dryness:
 Mercurius Vivus
 Phosphorus
Pressure And Heaviness:
 Kali Bichromicum

Ears:

Cold Feeling:
 Mercurius Vivus
Something In The Ears:
 Rhus Toxicodendron
Stopped Up:
 Bryonia
Wind Blowing In Ear:
 Rhus Toxicodendron

Extremities:

Bruised Feeling:
 Gelsemium Sempervirens
Cold Extremities:
 Gelsemium Sempervirens
 Mercurius Vivus
Cold Extremities With Hot Head And Back:
 Gelsemium Sempervirens

Cold And Tingling:
> Gelsemium Sempervirens

Numbness Of Hands And Feet In Fever:
> Lycopodium Clavatum

Tendons Too Tight:
> Pulsatilla Nigricans

Weakness In Muscles And Limbs:
> Gelsemium Sempervirens
> Phosphorus

Weakness And Tingling In Fingers:
> Natrum Muriaticum

Eyes:

Cold:
> Mercurius Vivus

Feel Bruised:
> Natrum Muriaticum

Feels Like Grit In Eye:
> Natrum Muriaticum

Feels Like Sand In Eyes:
> Aconitum Napellus
> Ferrum Phosphoricum
> Hepar Sulphuris Calcareum
> Kali Bichromicum

Inside Of Lids Feels Dry And Rough:
> Ferrum Phosphoricum

Pressure:
> Mercurius Vivus

Face:

Flashes Of Heat In Face:
> Mercurius Vivus

Head:

Cold Back Of Head:
> Phosphorus

Heavy:
> Aconitum Napellus
> Nux Vomica

Hot:
> Aconitum Napellus
> Belladonna
> Hot Head With Cold Feet:

Calcarea Carbonica
Hot Top Of Head With Cold Feet
Sulphur
Hot Head With Pale Face:
Calcarea Carbonica
Feels Like A Band Around The Head:
Gelsemium Sempervirens
Feels Like Head Will Burst:
Eupatorium Perfoliatum
Sulphur
Feels Like Head Is Being Squeezed:
Aconitum Napellus
Feels Like Head Is In A Vise:
Mercurius Vivus
Fullness:
Belladonna
Icy Chilliness:
Calcarea Carbonica
On Right Side:
Calcarea Carbonica
Nail In Top Of Head:
Nux Vomica
Pressure:
Nux Vomica
Sulphur
On Forehead:
Sulphur
Pulsation:
Aconitum Napellus
Tight Band Around Forehead:
Sulphur
Weight On Top Of Head:
Calcarea Carbonica
Larynx:
Ball In Larynx:
Sulphur
Speck In Larynx:
Belladonna
Swollen:
Sulphur

Mouth:
    Numbness And Tingling Of Lips:
        Natrum Muriaticum

Nose:
    Sensation Of A Hair In Left Nostril:
        Kali Bichromicum*

Stomach:
    Bloated, Swollen:
        Ferrum Phosphoricum
        Nux Vomica
    Emptiness:
        Gelsemium Sempervirens
    Heaviness Or Weight:
        Ferrum Phosphoricum
        Nux Vomica
    Lump After Eating:
        Natrum Muriaticum
    Stone In Stomach:
        Arsenicum Album

Throat:
    Ball In Throat:
        Sulphur
    Crumb In Throat:
        Hepar Sulphuris Calcareum
    Fish Bone In Throat:
        Hepar Sulphuris Calcareum
    Hair In Throat:
        Kali Bichromicum*
        Sulphur
    Lump In Throat:
        Allium Cepa
        Can't Be Swallowed:
            Gelsemium Sempervirens
        When Swallowing:
            Ferrum Phosphoricum
    Splinter In Throat:
        Hepar Sulphuris Calcareum*
        Sulphur

Tongue:
    Burnt Or Scalded:

Mercurius Vivus
Tip Feels Scalded:
Calcarea Carbonica
Lycopodium Clavatum
Hair On Tongue:
Kali Bichromicum*
Numbness And Tingling Of Tongue:
Natrum Muriaticum
Vascular:
Ice Or Boiling Water In Veins:
Arsenicum Album

Sleep:

Disturbances:
Groans And Talks:
Calcarea
Jerks:
Sulphur
Moans And Groans:
Belladonna
Rattling Breathing:
Kali Bichromicum
Sings:
Sulphur
Talks In Sleep:
Sulphur
Pulsatilla Nigricans
Yawning:
Allium Cepa
Hepar Sulphuris Calcareum
Dreams:
Aconitum Napellus
Dream Content:
Cliffs:
Allium Cepa
Anxious:
Calcarea Carbonica
Ferrum Phosphoricum
Lycopodium Clavatum
Mercurius Vivus
Phosphorus
Biting Dogs:
Mercurius Vivus
Confused:
Bryonia
Daily Business:
Bryonia
Dead People:
Calcarea Carbonica
Depressing:
Phosphorus

Dying:
    Gelsemium Sempervirens
Exertion:
    Rhus Toxicodendron
Frightful, Scary:
    Belladonna
    Calcarea Carbonica
    Mercurius Vivus
    Phosphorus
Gunshots:
    Mercurius Vivus
Happy:
    Sulphur
High Waves:
    Allium Cepa
Near Water:
    Allium Cepa
Robbers:
    Mercurius Vivus
Sick Persons:
    Calcarea Carbonica
Storms:
    Allium Cepa
Quarreling Leads To Happy Conversation:
    Ferrum Phosphoricum
Unfinished Business:
    Phosphorus
Violent, Horrible:
    Belladonna
    Phosphorus
Frequently:
    Calcarea Carbonica
Nightmares:
    Aconitum Napellus
    Belladonna
    Bryonia
Vivid:
    Calcarea Carbonica
    Sulphur
    Mercurius Vivus

Insomnia:
> Bryonia
> Hepar Sulphuris Calcareum
> Mercurius Vivus
> Natrum Muriaticum
> Sulphur
> Insomnia From Exhaustion:
>> Gelsemium Sempervirens
> Insomnia Late At Night:
>> Hepar Sulphuris Calcareum

Light Sleep:
> Gelsemium Sempervirens

Quality:
> Disturbed:
>> Lycopodium Clavatum

Position:
> Arms Crossed Over Abdomen:
>> Pulsatilla Nigricans
> Arms Raised Over Head:
>> Pulsatilla Nigricans
> Head High:
>> Eupatorium Perfoliatum
> On Back With Hand Under Head:
>> Aconitum Napellus
>> Arsenicum Album
> Side, Sleeping On Side Impossible:
>> Aconitum Napellus
>> Left Side, Sleeping On Left Side
>> Impossible:
>>> Eupatorium Perfoliatum
> Sitting Up:
>> Aconitum Napellus
>> Sitting Up Because Of Cough:
>>> Pulsatilla Nigricans

Prolonged Sleep:
> Hepar Sulphuris Calcareum

Restless:
> Aconitum Napellus
> Ferrum Phosphoricum
> Lycopodium Clavatum

Rhus Toxicodendron
Sleeps During the Day:
During The Day:
Pulsatilla Nigricans
During The Day But Sleepless At Night:
Phosphorus
Sleepy:
Sleepy Daytime:
Bryonia
Hepar Sulphuris Calcareum
Mercurius Vivus
Sulphur
Sleepy After Lunch:
Nux Vomica:
Sleepy Daytime And Early Evening:
Calcarea Carbonica
Sulphur
Sleepy Daytime, Restless Or Agitated At Night
Arsenicum Album
Unrefreshing:
Arsenicum Album
Bryonia
Kali Bichromicum
Wakes:
Frequently:
Sulphur
Time:
1:00 In The Morning:
Arsenicum Album
2:00 In The Morning:
Allium Cepa
2:00 In The Morning With
Headache And Nausea:
Kali Bichromicum
Between 2:00 And 5:00 In The Morning
Can't Sleep:
Sulphur
3:00 In The Morning:
Nux Vomica

3:00 In The Morning Wakes Up Feeling
Good, Falls Back Asleep And Wakes
Later In The Morning Feeling Badly:
> Nux Vomica

Too Early:
> Mercurius Vivus
> Too Early In The Morning And Sleeps
> Too Late:
>> Sulphur

With Anxiety:
> Aconitum Napellus

With Fright:
> Bryonia
> Pulsatilla Nigricans

With Palpitations And Sweating:
> Mercurius Vivus

From Slight Noise:
> Nux Vomica

Stomach:

Acid Reflux:
Nux Vomica
Clothing:
Tight Clothing, Pressure Of Clothing
Aggravates:
Ferrum Phosphoricum
Gelsemium Sempervirens
Wants Clothes Loosened:
Nux Vomica
Kali Bichromicum
Cramps (See Also Pain):
Belladonna
Nux Vomica
Sulphur
After Eating:
Eupatorium Perfoliatum
After Eating Only A Little:
Mercurius Vivus
Better:
Bending Backwards Or Forwards:
Belladonna
Cramps Extend To Back:
Belladonna

Diarrhea:
Lycopodium Clavatum
Summer Diarrhea:
Bryonia
Worse In The Afternoon:
Calcarea Carbonica

Diseases:
Stomach Flu:
Arsenicum Album*
Distended/Bloated:
Lycopodium Clavatum
Pulsatilla Nigricans
Sulphur

After A Small Amount Of Food:
Lycopodium Clavatum
Distended After A Meal:
Rhus Toxicodendron

Gas:
Belching:
Lycopodium Clavatum
Mercurius Vivus
Nux Vomica
After Eating:
Pulsatilla Nigricans
Frequent:
Arsenicum Album
Phosphorus
Frequent Sour Belching:
Calcarea Carbonica
Wants To Belch But Constriction
Prevents It:
Nux Vomica
With Bad Taste In Mouth:
Sulphur
With Stomach Pains After Eating:
Pulsatilla Nigricans
Gas (Without Belching):
Lycopodium Clavatum
Rhus Toxicodendron
Sulphur

Hiccups:
Mercurius Vivus
Violent Hiccups:
Natrum Muriaticum

Nausea:
Arsenicum Album
Belladonna
Rhus Toxicodendron
Sulphur
Alternating With Chills:

Hepar Sulphuris Calcareum
Due To Food Poisoning:
Arsenicum Album*
Phosphorus
Due To Stomach Flu
Arsenicum Album*
After Drinking:
Eupatorium Perfoliatum
After Eating:
Eupatorium Perfoliatum
Nux Vomica
In The Morning:
Hepar Sulphuris Calcareum
Feels As Though He Would Feel Better If
Only He Could Vomit:
Nux Vomica*
From:
Motion:
Lycopodium Clavatum
From Motion Especially In The
Morning:
Lycopodium Clavatum
Smell Of Food:
Eupatorium Perfoliatum
In The Morning:
Hepar Sulphuris Calcareum
Natrum Muriaticum
With:
Empty Hunger In The Morning:
Phosphorus
Faintness:
Bryonia
Pain In Stomach And Chest:
Mercurius Vivus
Yawning:
Bryonia
Worse In The Morning:
Nux Vomica

Pain:

Burning Pain:
>Sulphur

Burning And Gnawing Pain:
>Lycopodium Clavatum

Chronic Indigestion:
>Nux Vomica

Clutching Sensation Around The Belly Button:
>Belladonna

Eating:
>Better Cold Drinks And Food:
>>Phosphorus
>Food Lies In The Stomach Like A Stone:
>>Kali Bichromicum

Extends To Shoulders:
>Nux Vomica

Heartburn:
>After A Meal:
>>Kali Bichromicum
>Heartburn Pain May Extend To Back:
>>Kali Bichromicum
>Pain One And One-Half Hours After Eating:
>>Nux Vomica

With Nausea:
>Mercurius Vivus

Worse After Eating:
>Ferrum Phosphoricum

Pressure:

After A Meal:
>Sulphur

Pressure And Fullness:
>Rhus Toxicodendron

Pressure In Chest Or Stomach:
>Sulphur

In The Stomach After Eating Only A Little Food:
>Hepar Sulphuris Calcareum

Rumbling:

Lycopodium Clavatum

Pulsatilla Nigricans

Upset Stomach:
By Mild Food:
Kali Bichromicum
Worse Morning, Night, After A Meal:
Calcarea Carbonica

Vertigo And Bloated Stomach After Eating:
Rhus Toxicodendron

Vomiting:
Arsenicum Album
Belladonna
Sulphur
Due To Food Poisoning:
Arsenicum Album
Phosphorus
Eating:
After Any Attempt To Eat Or Drink:
Kali Bichromicum
As Soon As The Drink Is Warm In The
Stomach:
Phosphorus
Immediately After Eating:
Arsenicum Album
Retching:
Arsenicum Album
Spasms Of The Stomach With Empty
Retching:
Belladonna
Sour:
Calcarea Carbonica
What:
Bile:
Eupatorium Perfoliatum
Bright Yellow Water:
Kali Bichromicum
Mucus:
Mercurius Vivus

Undigested Food:
>> Ferrum Phosphoricum

When:
> Irregular Times:
>> Ferrum Phosphoricum

With Faintness:
> Bryonia

With Much Retching, Gagging, And Straining:
> Nux Vomica

With Yawning:
> Bryonia

Throat:

Better:
Holding Cold Water In Throat:
Lycopodium Clavatum*
Swallowing Liquid:
Cold:
Kali Bichromicum
Hot:
Kali Bichromicum
Warm:
Lycopodium Clavatum

Choking:
Wakes 2:00 In The Morning Choking:
Kali Bichromicum

Clears Throat Frequently:
Phosphorus

Color:
Red:
Belladonna*
Sulphur
Bluish Red:
Mercurius Vivus
Pulsatilla Nigricans
Dark Red:
Aconitum Napellus
Red Glottis:
Hepar Sulphuris Calcareum
Red Palate:
Ferrum Phosphoricum

Constricted/Tight:
Allium Cepa
Belladonna
Calcarea Carbonica
Gelsemium Sempervirens
Lycopodium Clavatum
Nux Vomica
Pulsatilla Nigricans
Constrictive, Swallowing:
Aconitum Napellus

Constrictive Swallowing So Liquids Come Out
Nose:
> Gelsemium Sempervirens
> Mercurius Vivus

Dry:

Allium Cepa
Belladonna*
Gelsemium Sempervirens
Kali Bichromicum
Mercurius Vivus
Phosphorus
Rhus Toxicodendron
Sulphur
Dry Red Throat, Worse Right Side:
> Belladonna*

Hot:

Allium Cepa
Gelsemium Sempervirens

Itchy:

Hepar Sulphuris Calcareum

Mucus:

Ferrum Phosphoricum
Rhus Toxicodendron
Sticky Mucus:
> Kali Bichromicum

Postnasal Drip:
> Natrum Muriaticum*
> Thick:
> > Kali Bichromicum

Pain:

Bruised:
> Rhus Toxicodendron

Burning:
> Aconitum Napellus
> Gelsemium Sempervirens
> Lycopodium Clavatum
> Sulphur

Chronic Sore Throat:
> Sulphur

Right Sided Or Moves Right To Left:
> Lycopodium Clavatum*

Sore:
> Anas Barbarae
> Nux Vomica

Sore Throat With Ulceration:
> Hepar Sulphuris Calcareum
> Kali Bichromicum

Sticking:
> Rhus Toxicodendron

Stinging:
> Aconitum Napellus
> Belladonna
> Pulsatilla Nigricans

Very Painful:
> Belladonna

Swallowing:
> When Swallowing:
> Aconitum Napellus
> Sticking Pain When Swallowing:
>> Rhus Toxicodendron
> Stitching Pain When Swallowing:
>> Calcarea Carbonica
>> Pulsatilla Nigricans

Worse:
> When Not Swallowing:
>> Nux Vomica
> When Swallowing:
>> Phosphorus
> Swallowing Empty:
>> Ferrum Phosphoricum
>> Mercurius Vivus
> Evening Or Afternoon:
>> Pulsatilla Nigricans
> Open Air:
>> Bryonia
> Right Side Of Throat:
>> Belladonna*

Raw:

Mercurius Vivus
Sulphur

Rough:
Gelsemium Sempervirens
Kali Bichromicum
Nux Vomica
Sulphur

Scraped:
Nux Vomica

Sensations (See Also "Sensation"   Section):
Lump In Throat, Cannot Be Swallowed:
Gelsemium Sempervirens
Plug In Throat:
Natrum Muriaticum
Nux Vomica
Sulphur
Plug In Throat Not Better From Swallowing:
Kali Bichromicum

Swallowing:
Difficult:
Arsenicum Album
Belladonna
Bryonia
Calcarea Carbonica
Gelsemium Sempervirens
Hepar Sulphuris Calcareum
Difficult, But Wants To Keep Swallowing:
Belladonna
Difficult Swallowing With Earache:
Gelsemium Sempervirens
Obstructed:
Lycopodium Clavatum

Swollen:
Rhus Toxicodendron
Nux Vomica
Pulsatilla Nigricans
Swollen, Bluish Red:
Mercurius Vivus
Swollen, Relieved By Cold:
Kali Bichromicum

Tickling:
>Hepar Sulphuris Calcareum
>Nux Vomica
>Tickling Back Of Throat:
>>Kali Bichromicum

Tingling:
>Aconitum Napellus

Tonsils:
>Color:
>>Red:
>>>Ferrum Phosphoricum
>>>Gelsemium Sempervirens
>>Purple:
>>>Sulphur
>Diseases:
>>Tonsillitis:
>>>Gelsemium Sempervirens
>>Recurrent Tonsillitis:
>>>Calcarea Carbonica
>Dry:
>>Aconitum Napellus
>>Belladonna
>>Bryonia
>>Ferrum Phosphoricum
>Inflamed:
>>Kali Bichromicum
>Sensitive:
>>Hepar Sulphuris Calcareum
>Itching And Tickling:
>>Gelsemium Sempervirens
>Sharp, Shooting Pain Left Tonsil:
>>Kali Bichromicum
>Sore:
>>Gelsemium Sempervirens
>Swollen/Enlarged:
>>Aconitum Napellus
>>Belladonna
>>Calcarea Carbonica
>>Ferrum Phosphoricum
>>Kali Bichromicum

Lycopodium Clavatum
Phosphorus
Sulfur
Ulcerative/Supporative:
Belladonna
Lycopodium Clavatum
Mercurius Vivus

Uvula:
Swollen:
Phosphorus
Weak Throat Muscles:
Gelsemium Sempervirens

Tongue:

Blisters:
Pulsatilla Nigricans
Edge Of Tongue:
Bryonia
Tip Of Tongue:
Lycopodium Clavatum
Color (See Also "Coated"):
Brownish:
Rhus Toxicodendron
Red:
Kali Bichromicum
Bright Red:
Arsenicum Album
Gelsemium Sempervirens
Rhus Toxicodendron
Pale:
Mercurius Vivus*
Red And Shiny:
Kali Bichromicum
Red At Edge And Tip:
Belladonna
Red, Triangular Tip Of Tongue:
Rhus Toxicodendron
White:
Arsenicum Album
Eupatorium Perfoliatum
White With Red Tip And Borders:
Sulphur
Coated (See Also "Color"):
Lycopodium Clavatum
Brown:
Bryonia
Kali Bichromicum
Lightly:
Gelsemium Sempervirens
Thickly Coated:
Nux Vomica
Wet And Coated:

Mercurius Vivus
White:
Aconitum Napellus
Bryonia
Rhus Toxicodendron
Nux Vomica
Phosphorus
Pulsatilla Nigricans
Yellow-White:
Aconitum Napellus
Bryonia
Gelsemium Sempervirens
Nux Vomica
Pulsatilla Nigricans

Cracked:
Arsenicum Album
Kali Bichromicum
Cracked Down Upper Center:
Mercurius Vivus

Dry:
Bryonia
Calcarea Carbonica
Gelsemium Sempervirens
Kali Bichromicum
Rhus Toxicodendron
Dry And Hot With An Aversion To Water:
Belladonna

Indented From Teeth:
Mercurius Vivus*

Pain:
Gelsemium Sempervirens
Sore:
Belladonna
Pain When Sticking Out Tongue:
Kali Bichromicum*

Qualities:
Smooth:
Kali Bichromicum
Furred, Trembling:
Gelsemium Sempervirens

Sensations (See Also "Sensations" Category):

Feels Thick:

Gelsemium Sempervirens

Tongue Raw:

Gelsemium Sempervirens

Numb:

Gelsemium Sempervirens

Tip Of Tongue Tingles:

Aconitum Napellus

Paralyzed Tongue:

Gelsemium Sempervirens

Swollen:

Swollen And Red:

Mercurius Vivus*

Swollen and Pale:

Mercurius Vivus*

Ulcers:

Mercurius Vivus*

Natrum Muriaticum*

Worse:

Bathing:
Washing:
Sulphur
Clothing:
Tight Clothes:
Lycopodium Clavatum
Too Many Coverings:
Pulsatilla Nigricans
Undressing:
Hepar Sulphuris Calcareum
Rhus Toxicodendron
Warmly Wrapped Up:
Bryonia
Environment:
Before And During A Thunderstorm:
Phosphorus
Change Of Weather:
Phosphorus
Cold Air:
Lycopodium Clavatum
Cold Damp Weather:
Kali Bichromicum
Cold Dry Weather:
Hepar Sulphuris Calcareum
Cold Dry Wind:
Aconitum Napellus
Cold, Dry, and Windy Weather:
Nux Vomica
Cold Fresh Air:
Rhus Toxicodendron
Cold Water:
Calcarea Carbonica
Cold Wet Air After Rain:
Rhus Toxicodendron
Cold Wet Weather:
Calcarea Carbonica
Cold Wind:
Allium Cepa

Belladonna
Hepar Sulphuris Calcareum
Cool Surroundings:
Belladonna
Cool Weather:
Damp And Cold Weather:
Mercurius Vivus
Sulphur
Damp Weather:
Gelsemium Sempervirens
Drafts:
Arsenicum Album
Belladonna
Wet Weather:
Arsenicum Album
Eye Symptoms Worse In Open Air:
Euphrasia Officinalis
Fog:
Gelsemium Sempervirens
Fresh Air:
Natrum Muriaticum
Getting Feet Wet:
Allium Cepa
Getting Wet (But Better Wet Weather):
Nux Vomica
Hot Air:
Lycopodium Clavatum
Hot Room:
Gelsemium Sempervirens
Humidity:
Gelsemium Sempervirens
Pulsatilla Nigricans
Indoor Drafts:
Arsenicum Album
Indoors:
Euphrasia Officinalis
Least Draft:
Hepar Sulphuris Calcareum
May Be Either Better Or Worse At Seaside Or
Near The Sea:

Ferrum Phosphoricum
Natrum Muriaticum
Open Air:
Arsenicum Album
Eye Symptoms Are Worse In Open Air:
Euphrasia Officinalis
Open Air/Outdoors:
Arsenicum Album*
Ferrum Phosphoricum
Kali Bichromicum
Nux Vomica
Rainy Weather:
Mercurius Vivus
Stuffy Or Warm Room:
Aconitum Napellus
Sun:
Gelsemium Sempervirens
Very Cold Weather:
Mercurius Vivus
Very Hot Weather:
Mercurius Vivus
Sulphur
Warm Or Stuffy Room:
Allium Cepa
Warm Room:
Bryonia
Pulsatilla Nigricans
When Snow Is Melting:
Kali Bichromicum
Windy Weather:
Euphrasia Officinalis
Nux Vomica

Food and Drink:
After Eating:
Pulsatilla Nigricans
Alcohol:
Kali Bichromicum
Sulphur
Coffee:
Nux Vomica

Cold Drinks:
    Arsenicum Album
    Ferrum Phosphoricum
Cold Food:
    Arsenicum Album
    Nux Vomica
Cold Water:
    Aconitum Napellus
    Nux Vomica
Drinking:
    Arsenicum Album
    Belladonna
Eating:
    Arsenicum Album
    Ferrum Phosphoricum
    Nux Vomica
Eggs:
    Anas Barbarae
Fasting:
    Phosphorus
Gets Sick From Skipped Meals:
    Lycopodium Clavatum
Milk:
    Anas Barbarae
Overeating:
    Lycopodium Clavatum
Rich Food:
    Pulsatilla Nigricans
Room Temperature Food And Drinks:
    Lycopodium Clavatum
Spicy Food:
    Nux Vomica
Stimulants:
    Nux Vomica
Warm Food And Drink:
    Phosphorus
Wine:
    Nux Vomica
Cold Food And Drinks:
    Lycopodium Clavatum

Hot And Cold:
  Extremes Of Temperature:
      Natrum Muriaticum
  Going From Hot To Cold And Vice Versa:
      Phosphorus
  Cold:
      Hepar Sulphuris Calcareum*
      Rhus Toxicodendron
      Cold Applications:
          Rhus Toxicodendron
      Cold Cloth:
          Rhus Toxicodendron
      Getting Cold:
          Hepar Sulphuris Calcareum
      Severe Cold:
          Sulphur
  Heat:
      Gelsemium Sempervirens
      Ferrum Phosphoricum
      Getting Hot:
          Natrum Muriaticum
      Hot Room:
          Gelsemium Sempervirens
          Warmth:
              Euphrasia Officinalis
          Warmth Of Bed:
              Mercurius Vivus
Light:
  Arsenicum Album
  Belladonna
  Euphrasia Officinalis
  Nux Vomica
  Sunlight:
      Belladonna
Mental:
  Anxiety:
      Calcarea
      Nux Vomica
  Bad News:
      Gelsemium Sempervirens

Emotions:
>	Gelsemium Sempervirens

Excitement:
>	Gelsemium Sempervirens

Thinking Of Ailment:
>	Gelsemium Sempervirens

Motion:

Jarring The Bed:
>	Belladonna

Motion:
>	Ferrum Phosphoricum
>	Hepar Sulphuris Calcareum
>	Nux Vomica

Movement:
>	Arsenicum Album
>	Belladonna
>	Bryonia
>	Eupatorium Perfoliatum

Stooping:
>	Kali Bichromicum

Walking:
>	Ferrum Phosphoricum

Noise:

Arsenicum Album
Belladonna
Natrum Muriaticum
Nux Vomica

Loud Noise:
>	Ferrum Phosphoricum

Music:
>	Natrum Muriaticum

Sudden Noise:
>	Natrum Muriaticum

Odors:

Tobacco Smoke:
>	Aconitum Napellus
>	Gelsemium Sempervirens
>	Lycopodium Clavatum
>	Nux Vomica

Overwork:

Physical:
>> Calcarea

Study:
>> Sulphur

Exertion:
>> Hepar Sulphuris Calcareum
>> Nux Vomica
>> Mental Exertion:
>>> Calcarea
>>> Nux Vomica
>>> Phosphorus
>> Physical Exertion:
>>> Ferrum Phosphoricum
>>> Phosphorus

Position:

Bending Forward:
>> Belladonna

Lying Down:
>> Belladonna
>> Euphrasia Officinalis
>> Natrum Muriaticum
>> Lying In Bed:
>>> Ferrum Phosphoricum
>> Lying On Back:
>>> Eupatorium
>> Lying On Side:
>>> Lying On Left Side:
>>>> Natrum Muriaticum
>>> Lying On Right Side:
>>>> Aconitum Napellus
>>>> Arsenicum Album
>>>> Belladonna
>>>> Ferrum Phosphoricum
>>>> Lycopodium Clavatum
>>>> Rhus Toxicodendron
>> Lying With Raised Head:
>>> Arsenicum Album

Sitting:
>> Prolonged Sitting:
>>> Sulphur

Sitting In One Position For A Long
Time:
    Rhus Toxicodendron
Standing:
    Sulphur
Stooping:
    Belladonna

Pressure:
    Belladonna
    Hepar Sulphuris Calcareum
    Natrum Muriaticum

Rest:
    Ferrum Phosphoricum
    Rhus Toxicodendron

Sleep:
    Natrum Muriaticum
    Sleeping In Bed:
        Lycopodium Clavatum
    Interrupted:
        Aconitum Napellus
    Oversleeping:
        Sulphur
    Warmth Of Bed:
        Mercurius Vivus
        Sulphur

Sweating:
    Mercurius Vivus
    Getting Overheated:
        Pulsatilla Nigricans

Time:
    Afternoon:
        Belladonna
        Fatigue Every Afternoon Between 4:00
        And 5:00:
            Gelsemium Sempervirens
    During Full Moon:
        Calcarea Carbonica
    Evening:
        Phosphorus
        Pulsatilla Nigricans

Evening Until Midnight:
    Hepar Sulphuris Calcareum
Toward Evening:
    Allium Cepa
4:00-8:00 In The Evening:
    Lycopodium Clavatum
7:00 In The Evening:
    Rhus Toxicodendron
8:00-9:00 In The Evening:
    Nux Vomica
Fever Peaks At 9:00 In The Evening:
    Belladonna
Midnight:
    Sulphur
    After Midnight:
        Aconitum Napellus
        Arsenicum Album
        Nux Vomica
    Before Midnight:
    Just Before Midnight:
        Arsenicum Album
    Between Midnight And 2:00 Or 3:00 In
    The Morning:
        Arsenicum Album
Morning:
    Kali Bichromicum
    Nux Vomica
    Sulphur
    Morning And Evening:
        Hepar Sulphuris Calcareum
    After 1:00 In The Morning:
        Arsenicum Album
    2:00-3:00 In The Morning:
        Kali Bichromicum
    3:00 In The Morning:
        Kali Bichromicum
    3:00-4:00 In The Morning:
        Ferrum Phosphoricum
    10:00 In The Morning:
        Gelsemium Sempervirens

10:00-11:00 In The Morning:
Natrum Muriaticum
11:00 In The Morning:
Sulphur
Chills Worse 7:00-9:00 In The Morning:
Eupatorium
Fever Peaks At 8:00 In The Morning:
Belladonna
Stuffiness Worse In The Morning:
Euphrasia Officinalis
Night:
Aconitum Napellus
Belladonna
Euphrasia Officinalis
Ferrum Phosphoricum
Mercurius Vivus
Pulsatilla Nigricans
Sulphur
Nasal Discharge Worse At Night:
Euphrasia Officinalis
Noon:
Sulphur
Seasons:
Autumn:
Mercurius Vivus
Spring (They Tend To Get Colds):
Sulphur
Twilight:
Phosphorus
Waking:
Lycopodium Clavatum

Touch:
Hepar Sulphuris Calcareum
Kali Bichromicum
Natrum Muriaticum
Nux Vomica

APPENDIX

List Of Twenty Questions
To Ask About Colds And Flu

    1. *What was he doing when the cold came on?* Had he been chilled, out in the wind, under some physical or emotional stress? Overworked? Had a major disappointment? Did he just suffer an injury or have surgery? Was there a change in the weather? Did he eat food that could have been tainted? In other words, do you feel anything unusual happened to him that could have made him susceptible to the cold or flu?

    2. *How is his state of mind?* How are his memory and concentration? Is there a type of thinking he prefers? Conceptual, abstract? Is he artistic or mechanically minded? Is he unusually fearful, anxious, depressed, or angry? Is he afraid? If so, of what? How is his temper? Has he been startling easily? Has he been sad? If so, what time of day does he seem to be worse or better? There is a great temptation to blame emotional states on circumstance, such as, "Well, he has been sad, but his pet died, or his friend moved away. . ." You have to use your own judgment on how much circumstance has to do with the patient's emotional state. I usually look for excessive patterns of thought—maybe the dog did die, but has he been crying overmuch? Yes, he is awaiting important test results—but is he anxious out of proportion to the event?

    3. *Any head symptoms?* How does his head feel? Does he have vertigo (dizziness)? If so, what time of day does it happen? What makes the vertigo better? What makes it worse? Does he have a headache? If so, where does it hurt on his head? What does it feel like? What makes the headache better or worse? Is it worse at a certain time of day? Is his scalp sore?

    4. *Is his face any different?* Is his face swollen, pale, red, and if so, is it on both sides equally? Does he have circles under his eyes? Does his face hurt? If so, where?

    5. *Any eye symptoms?* Are they swollen, red, itchy, tearing? If they are tearing, do the tears burn? How do his eyes

feel when they are moved and used? Are his pupils dilated? Are they sensitive to light? Are there any disturbances of vision, such as specks? When are the eyes better or worse? What makes them better or worse?

6. *How do his ears feel?* Does he have roaring or other sounds in his ears? Is he sensitive to noise? Are his ears hot or red? Is there pus in his ears? Does the ear pain travel down the neck or anywhere else? Does he feel like he has fluid in his ears?

7. *How does his nose feel?* Does he have a nasal discharge? How does the nasal discharge smell to him? What color (green, yellow, clear) is it? What consistency is it? (ropy, thick, thin, watery). Are both nostrils equally stuffy, running, or blocked? Does the discharge alternate between being runny and blocked? Does the discharge burn the nostrils or the upper lip? How does his nose feel? Is his nose sore? What color is the outside of his nose? Is he sneezing, and does the sneezing relieve his stuffiness?

8. *How are his mouth and tongue?* Is his tongue coated? Does it have any cracks in it? Is it flabby, showing the imprint of the teeth? Does he have mouth ulcers? Are his mouth and tongue sore? Are his lips dry or cracked?

9. *Does he have a sore throat?* Is his throat red, white, swollen? Does his throat feel constricted? Is it worse swallowing, worse when he doesn't swallow, or is it sore all the time? *How* does it hurt? Scraped, tingling, raw? Any sensation of a lump, splinter, or hair in his throat? How much does it hurt? Are the throat muscles so constricted that liquids come out of his nose?

10. *And his larynx?* Is he hoarse? Does it hurt in the larynx when he coughs or breathes in? Is he hoarse at a certain time of day? Is he more hoarse or less hoarse when he talks a while? Does he have mucus in his larynx? What does his voice sound like?

11. *Ask about his neck and back.* Are they painful or stiff? If so, where? What kind of neck or back pain does he have? Throbbing, aching, etc.? What makes the pain better or worse? Does he feel like the muscles of his back are sore, or does it feel like it's the bones that are aching? Are his lymph nodes swollen?

12. *Any Chest Symptoms?* How well is he breathing? Is he short of breath? Is his chest burning or constricted? Does he have any chest pain?

13. *Is he coughing?* If so, is it dry, wet, hacking, painful in his chest or head? Is it worse or better lying down? When he

coughs something up, what does it look like? Is there a time of day when the cough is worse or better? What makes the cough worse or better? Does the cough make him choke, retch, or vomit? Is he coughing up blood?

14. *Extremities?* How do his arms, legs, hands, and feet feel? Are they cold or hot? Are they stiff or sore? Is he having any muscle cramps, numbness, or tingling? Do his arms or legs fall asleep easily?

15. *Does he have stomach trouble?* Does he have cramps, belching, nausea, or diarrhea? If he has cramps or nausea, is it worse after he eats or before he eats? What makes the cramps better or worse? Has he been vomiting? Does he have any appetite? If he has diarrhea, what is it like? (Watery, unusual color, etc.) Does the diarrhea burn? Does his stomach feel bloated or heavy?

16. *What about food?* Is he thirsty? What does he want to eat or drink? What does he definitely *not* want to eat or drink? What disagrees with him, gives him gas or stomach pains or diarrhea? Does his food taste unusual? (Please note: an *aggravation* is a stomach upset from eating a particular food. An *aversion* is an avoidance of a particular food; he doesn't want to eat it, but if he did, it wouldn't make him physically ill. Of course, you can have a food that you have both an aversion to which gives you an aggravation. It is important to make the distinction when taking a case.)

17. *How is he sleeping?* Has he been restless, waking up in the night? If so, what time? Has he had any nightmares or dreams that he remembers? What position does he sleep in?

18. *Is he running a fever?* How high has it been? Does he have chills? How do the chills and fever come on? Is he perspiring, and if so, where?

19. *What makes him feel better?* Does he want to be left alone, have a hot bath, bundle up, be outdoors, have company, eat, not eat? What time of day does he feel better?

20. *What makes him feel worse?* Is he worse after he eats, after talking, after not sleeping, when he first gets up? Are there drinks or food that makes him feel worse? What time of day does he feel worse?

21. *General questions?* Did the illness come on suddenly or gradually? Do the symptoms start in the chest and go up to the

nose or vice versa? Do the symptoms alternate, such as the nasal discharge alternating with headache? Do they seem to be left or right sided, or move from right to left? Which side is worse? Are his senses dull or hyperacute? Does he have sensations like something blowing on him? Are there changes in behavior? Does he have any unusual postures? Coughing with his hand on his chest, sleeps sitting up? Do tight clothes bother him? Is he trembling or shaking? Do any of the pains shift from one part to another?

Use phrases such as "what else?" or "anything else?" to get more information. Asking questions like, "Is your throat sore?" to elicit a "yes or no" answer is not as productive and often leads to less information. Try for a mix of different questions to get all the information you can.

															Extras
Aconitum															
Allium Cepa															
Anas Barbar.															
Arsenicum															
Belladonna															
Bryonia															
Calcarea Carb															
Eupatorium															
Euphrasia															
Ferrum Phos															
Gelsemium															
Hepar Sulph															
Influenzinum															
Kali Bichrom.															
Lycopodium															
Mercury															
Natrum Mur															
Nux Vomica															
Phosphorus															
Pulsatilla															
Rhus Tox															
Sulphur															

Homeopathy Resources

Information On Study Groups, Membership, Newsletter:

National Center For Homeopathy
801 North Fairfax St., Suite 306
Alexandria, VA 22314
(703) 548-7790

Pharmacy, Books, And Information:

Boiron
98C W. Cochran St.
Simi Valley, CA 93065
1-800-Blu Tube

Dolisos
3014 Rigel Ave.
Las Vegas, NV 89102
1-800-DOLISOS

Hahnemann Laboratories
1940 Fourth Street
San Rafael, CA 94901
1-888-427-6422

Homeopathy Overnight
929 Shelburne Ave.
Absecon, NJ 08201
1-800-ARNICA-30

Luyties
P.O. Box 8080
Richford, VT 05476
1-800-325-8080

Homeopathic Educational Services
2124 Kittredge St.
Berkeley, CA 94704
Inquiries/Catalogs: 510-649-0294
Orders: 1-800-359-9051

Standard Homeopathic Co.
210 West 131 St.
Box 61067
Los Angeles, C: 90061
1-800-624-9659

(Remedy Order Department For Standard Homeopathic
     Company)

Arrowroot Standard Direct
83 East Lancaster Avenue
Paoli, PA 19301
1-800-234-8879

For those of you who want to delve deeper into homeopathy,
this company has computer software to help you find the
right remedy for a case. They also have other educational
resources for homeopathy.

Kent Homeopathic Associates
710 Mission Ave.
San Rafael, CA 94901
(415) 457-0678

Bibliography

Anderson, David, M.D., Dale Buegel, M.D. and Dennis Chernin. *Homeopathic Remedies For Physicians, Laymen, and Therapists.* Homesdale: Himalayan Institute Press, 1991.

Bailey, Philip M. M.D. *Homeopathic Psychology.* Berkeley, California: North Atlantic Books, 1995.

Bellavite, Paolo, MD and Andrea Signorini, MD. *Homeopathy: A Frontier In Medical Science.* Berkeley, CA: North Atlantic Books, 1995.

Boericke, William, MD. *Materia Medica.* Santa Rosa, CA: Boericke and Tafel, 1927.

Clarke, J. H., MD. *A Clinical Repertory To The Dictionary of Materia Medica.* New Delhi, India: B. Jain Publishers, reprinted 1992.

Clarke, John Henry, MD. *A Dictionary of Practical Materia Medica, Volumes 1, 2, and 3.* New Delhi: B. Jain Publishers, reprinted 1992.

Coulter, Catherine R. *Portraits of Homeopathic Medicines, Volumes 1 & 2*: Berkeley, CA: North Atlantic Books, 1988.

Gibson, Douglas. *Studies of Homeopathic Remedies.* Beaconsfield, Bucks, England: Beaconsfield, 1991.

Gibson, D.M. *First Aid Homeopathy.* London: The British Homeopathic Association, 1991.

Hadley, Rima. *A Homeopathic Love Story.* Berkeley, CA: North Atlantic Books, 1990.
Hahnemann, Samuel. Organon of Medicine. Los Angeles: J. P. Tarcher, Inc., translation ©1982 by the Hahnemann Foundation.

Hammond, Christopher. *The Complete Family Guide To Homeopathy*. New York: Penguin, 1995.

Harrison, Shiela. *Help Your Child With Homeopathy*. Ashgrove Press, 1996.

Jonas, Wayne B., MD and Jennifer Jacobs, MD. *Healing With Homeopathy*. New York: Warner Books, 1996.

Kaufman, Martin. *Homeopathy In America: the Rise and Fall of a Medical Heresy*. Baltimore: Johns Hopkins Press, 1971.

Kent, James Tyler, MD. *Lectures on Homeopathic Philosophy*. Berkeley, CA: North Atlantic Books, originally published in 1900.

Koehler, Gerhard. *Handbook of Homeopathy*. Rochester, Vermont: Healing Arts Press, 1989.

Lockie, Andrew, MD, and Dr. Nicole Geddes, MD. *Homeopathy: The Principles and Practice of Treatment*. New York: Darling Kindersley, 1995.

Mitchell, G. Ruthven. *Homeopathy*. London: W.H. Allen: 1975.

Murphy, Robin, N.D. *Homeopathic Medical Repertory*: Pagosa Springs, CA: Hahnemann Academy Of North America: 1993.

Panos, Maesimond, MD and Jane Heimlich: *Homeopathic Medicine at Home*. New York: J.P. Tarcher, St. Martin's Press, 1980.

Perry, Edmond L., MD. *Luyties Homeopathic Practice*. St. Louis, MO: Formur, 1974.

Roberts, Herbert A, MD, *The Principles and Art Of Cure By Homeopathy*. Kent: Health Science Press, Whitstable Litho, 1976.
Shadman, Alonzo J. *Who Is Your Doctor and Why:* Connecticut: Keats Publishing, 1980.

Ullman, Dana, N.D. *Consumer's Guide to Homeopathy*. New York: Jeremy P. Tarcher, Putnum, 1995.

Ullman, Dana, N.D. *Homeopathic Medicine For Children and Infants*. New York: Jeremy P. Tarcher, 1992.

Ullman, Dana, N.D. *Homeopathy: Medicine For the 21st Century*. Berkeley: North Atlantic Books, 1988.

Ullman, Robert, ND and Judyth Reichenberger Ullman, ND. *Homeopathic Self-Care: The Quick and Easy Guide For the Whole Family.* Rocklin, CA: Prima Publishing, 1997.

Vithoulkas, George. *The Science of Homeopathy*. New York: Grove Press, 1980.

Index To
Cold And Flu Repertory

www.ingramcontent.com/pod-product-compliance
Lightning Source LLC
Chambersburg PA
CBHW021848020426
42334CB00013B/234